The FART BOOK

A BOOK FOR CHILDREN TO ENJOY AND LEARN ABOUT THE BODY'S GAS, FLATULENCE, AND OTHER STINKY FACTS

STORY AND ILLUSTRATION BY MARK BACERA

COPYRIGHT © 2020 by ROUNDED SPECS PUBLISHING, LLC., ISBN 978-1-952343-00-1

This book is for:

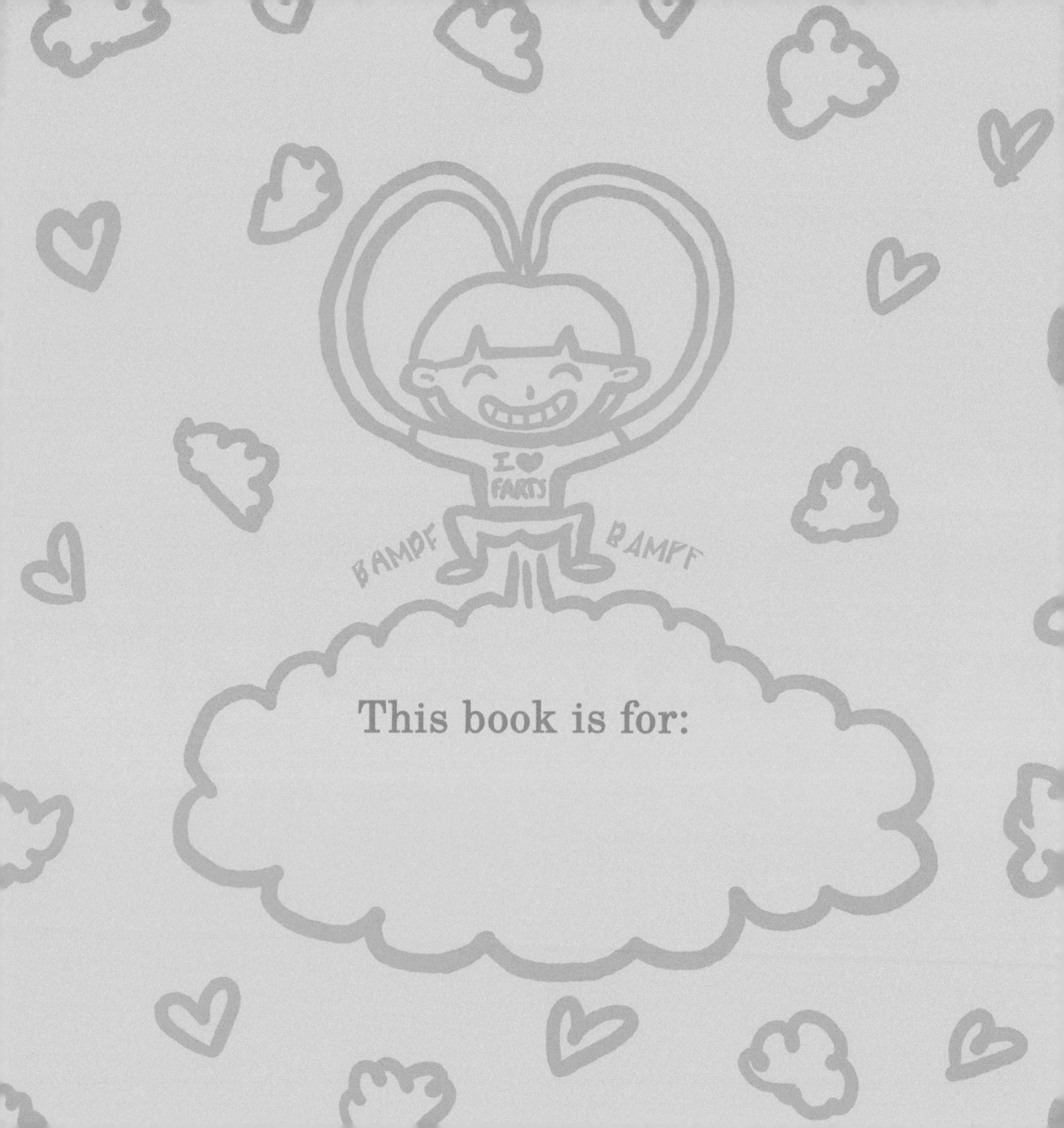

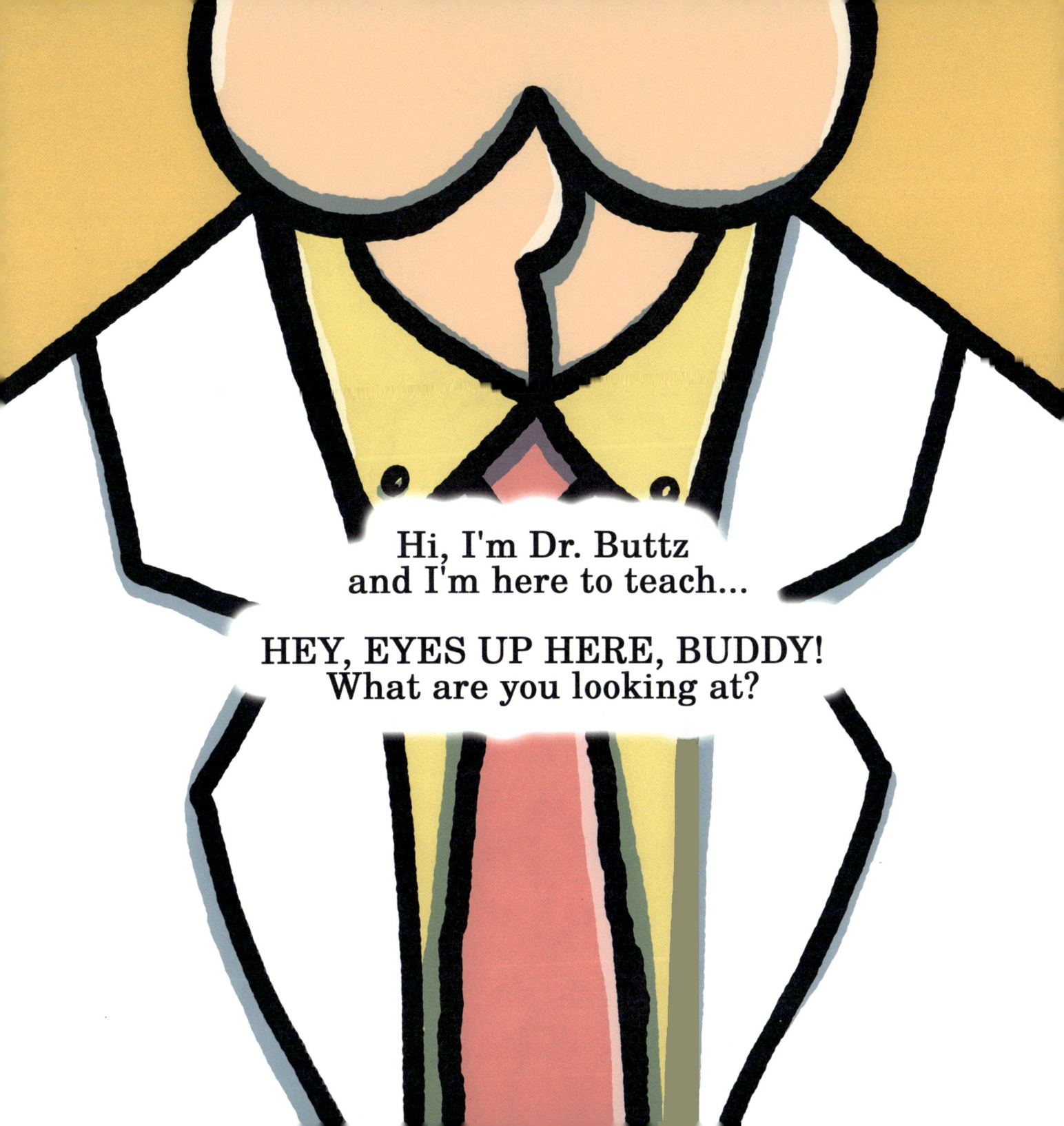

Hi, I'm Dr. Buttz
and I'm here to teach...

HEY, EYES UP HERE, BUDDY!
What are you looking at?

That's better!

I'm Dr. Buttz and I'm here
to teach you about farts.

So, let me tell you *all* about our stinky friends
in a *little* rhyme I made...

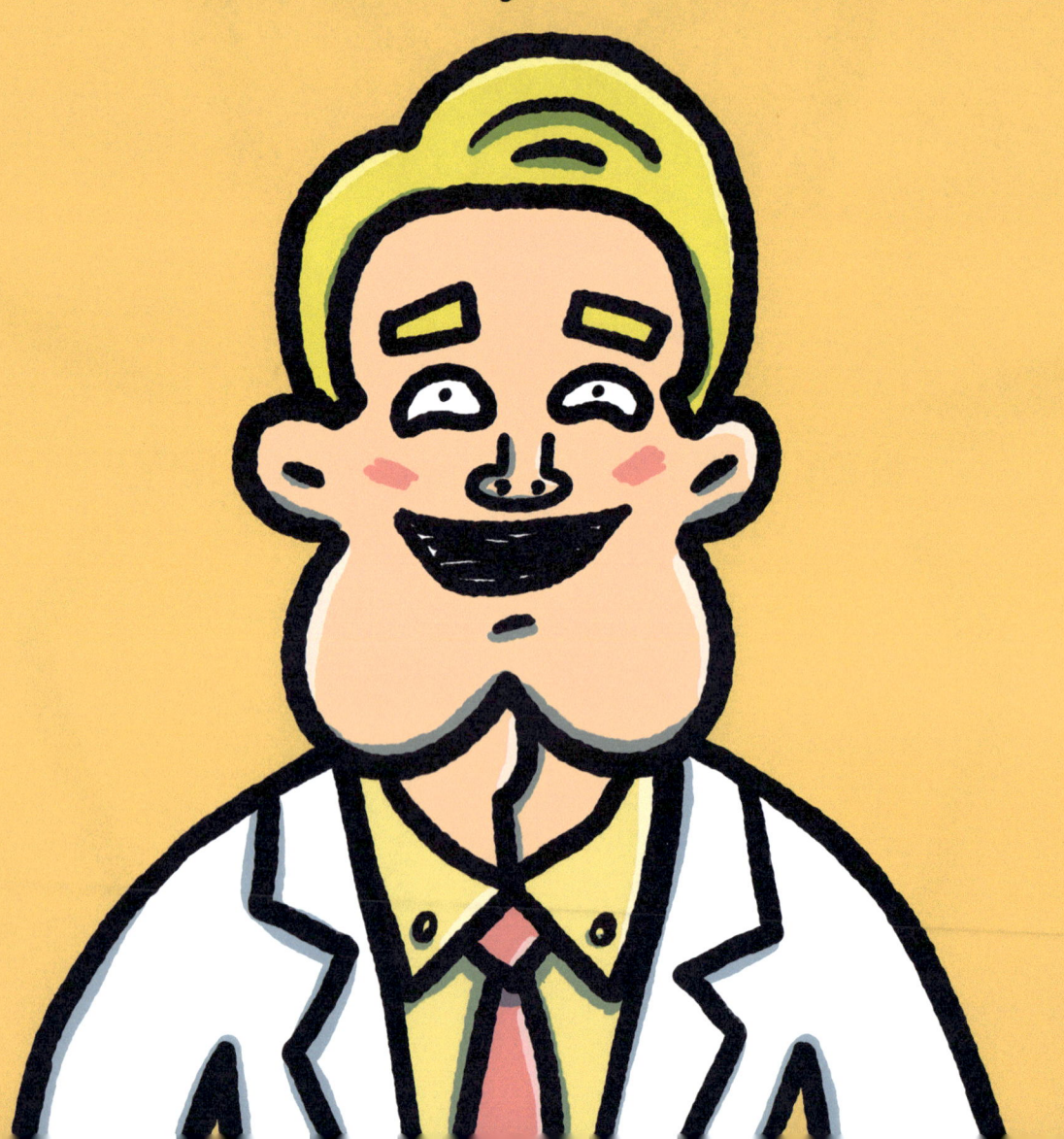

Some farts are like...

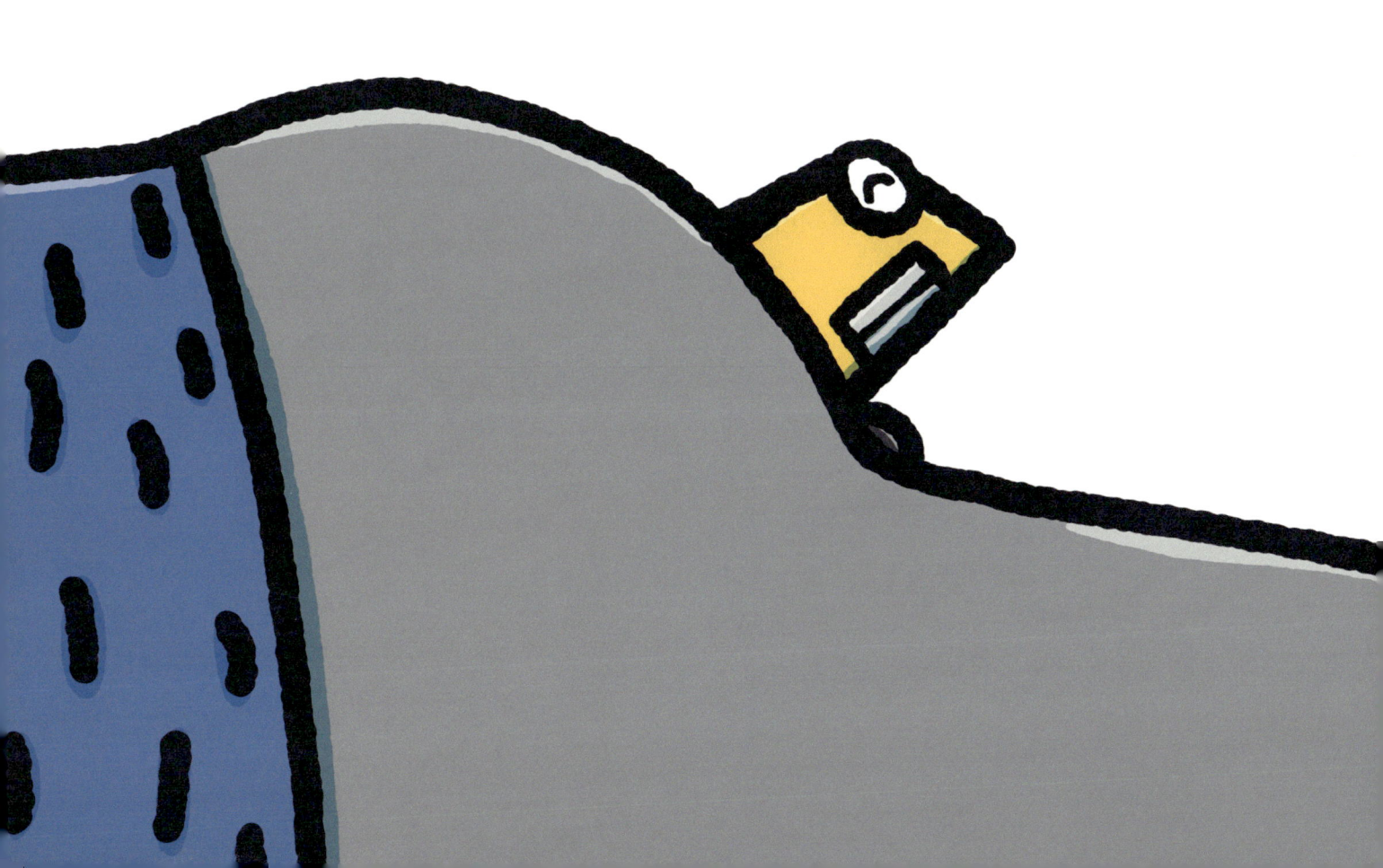

CARS!

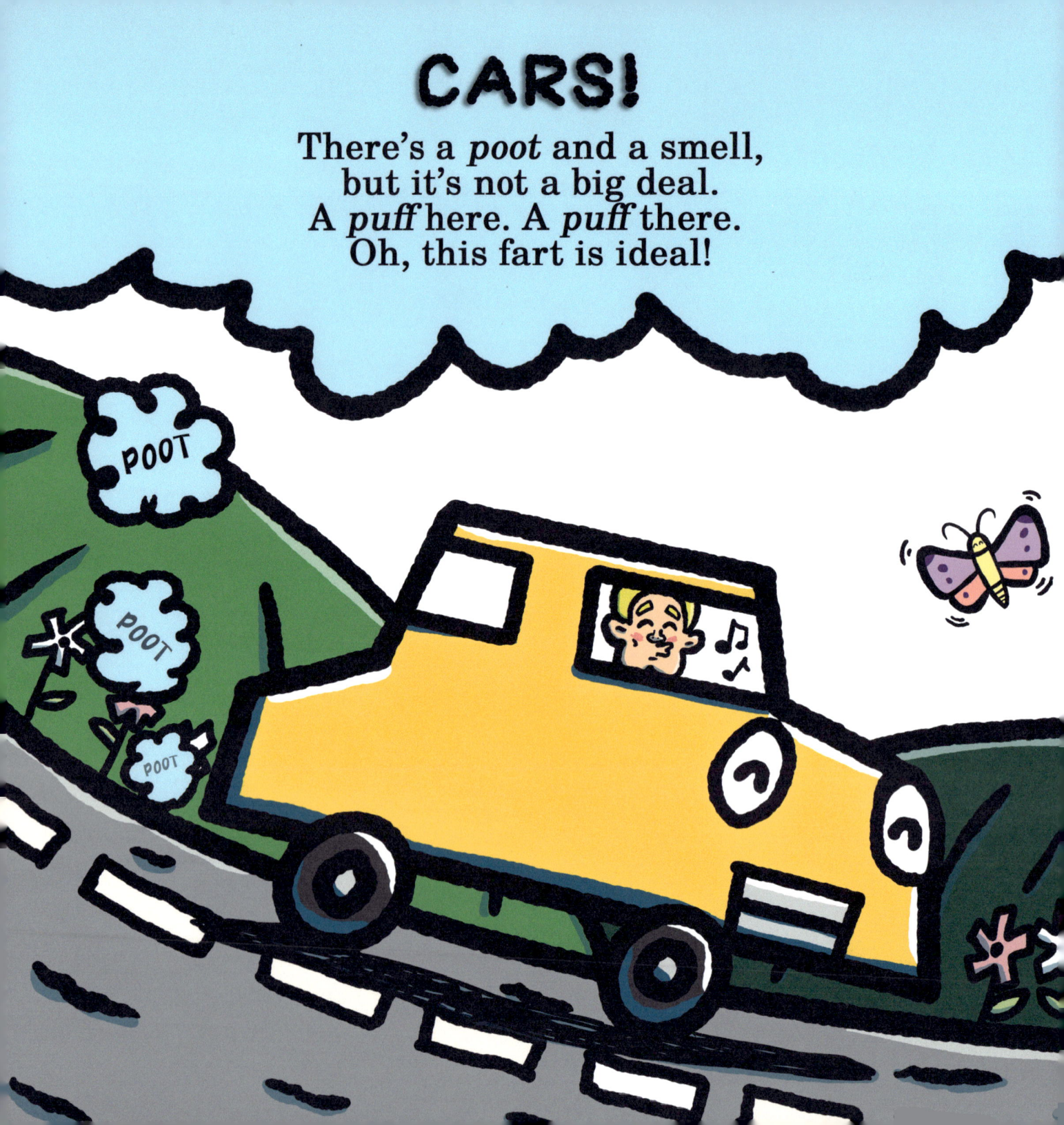

There's a *poot* and a smell,
but it's not a big deal.
A *puff* here. A *puff* there.
Oh, this fart is ideal!

Some farts are like...

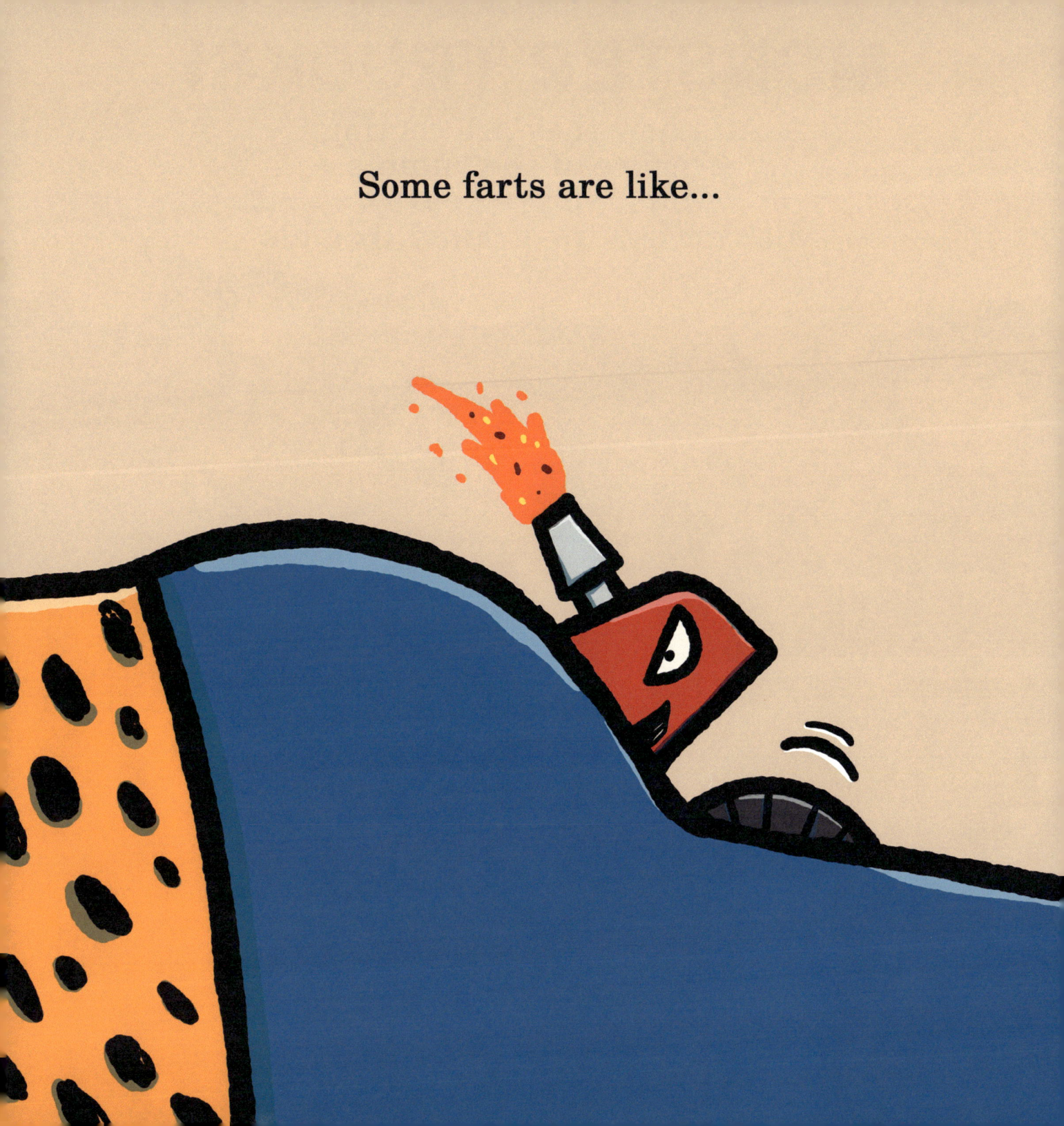

MONSTER TRUCKS!

All know they are coming,
because of the rumble.
And if you're nearby,
you can feel the ground tremble.

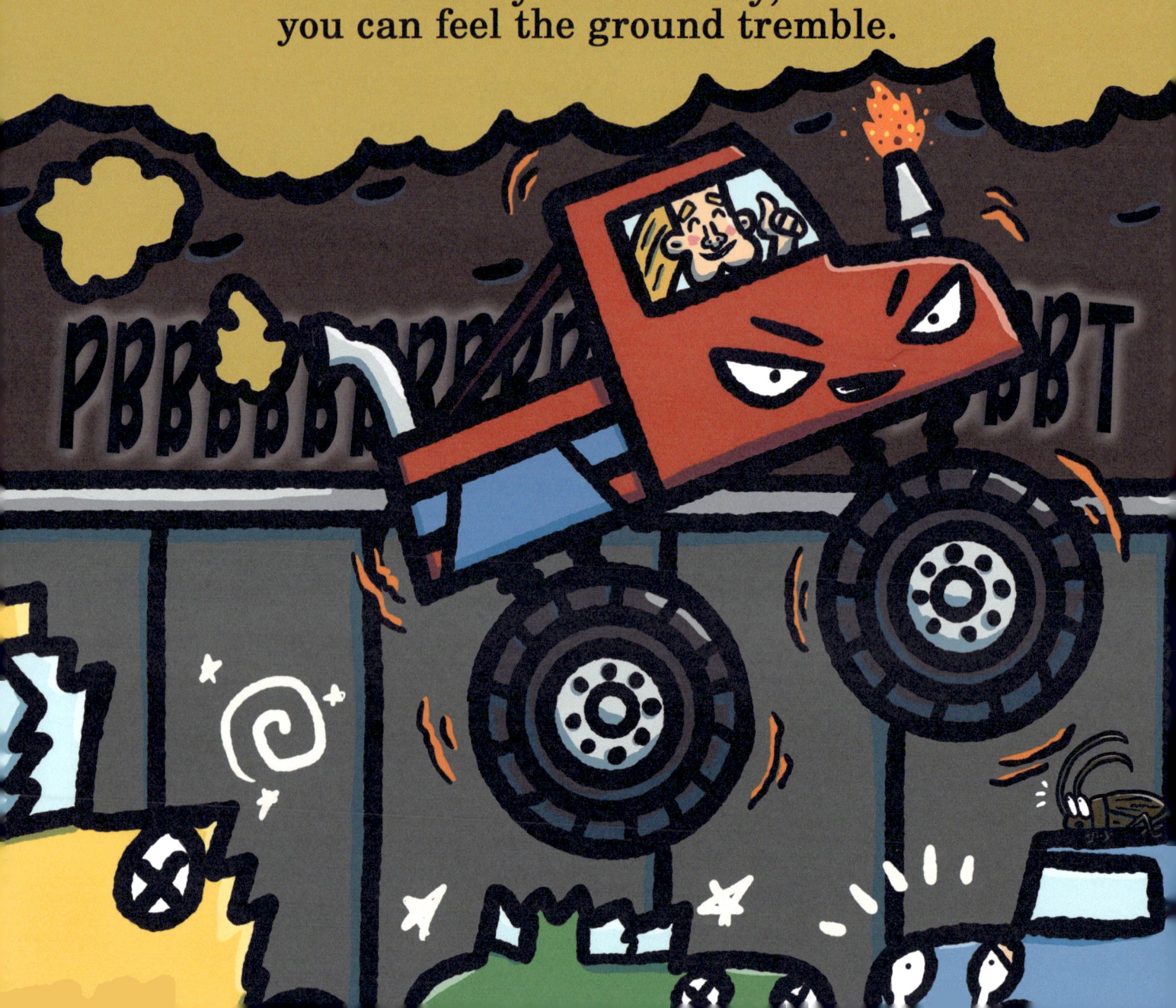

Some farts are like...

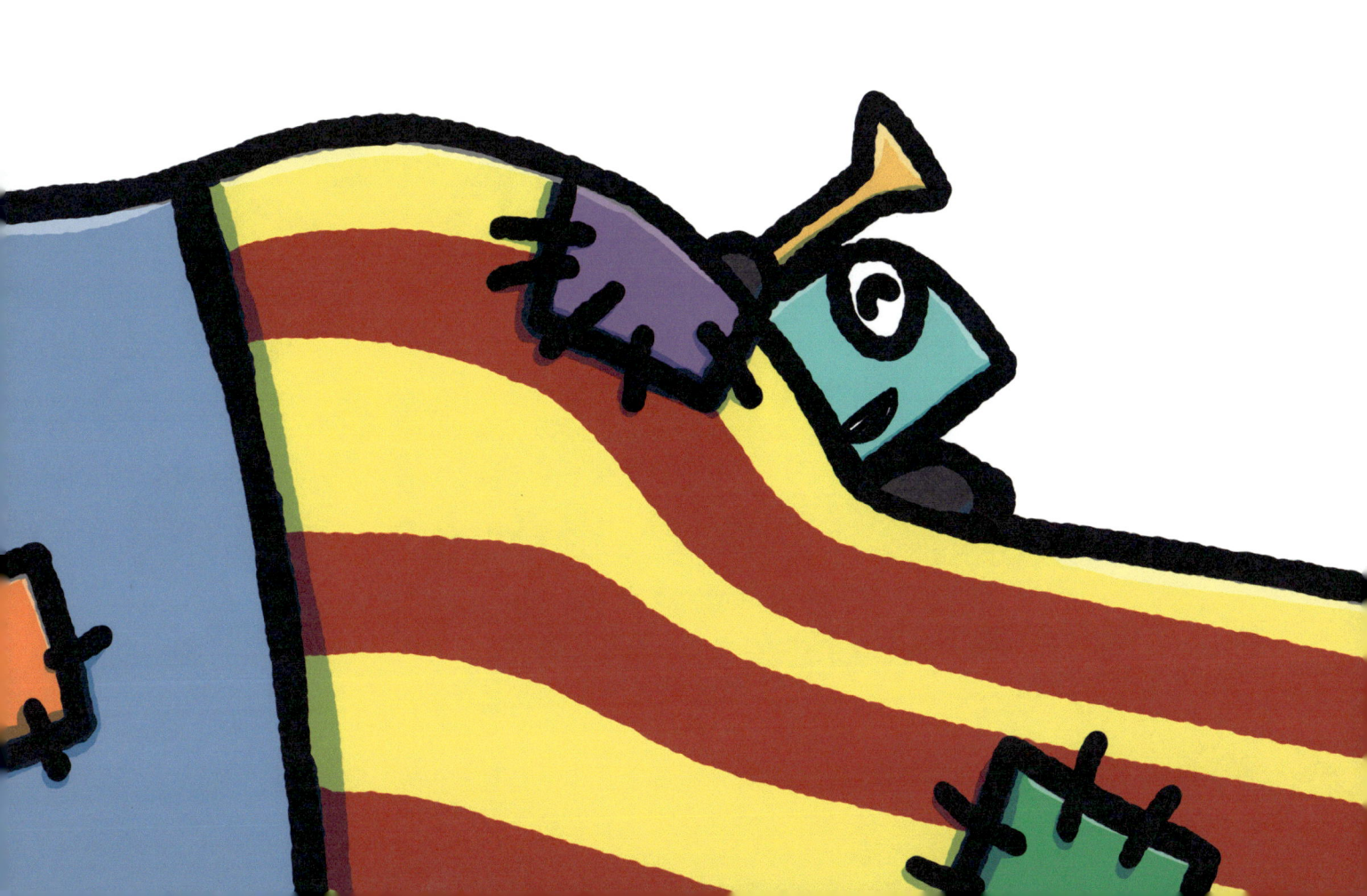

CLOWN CARS!

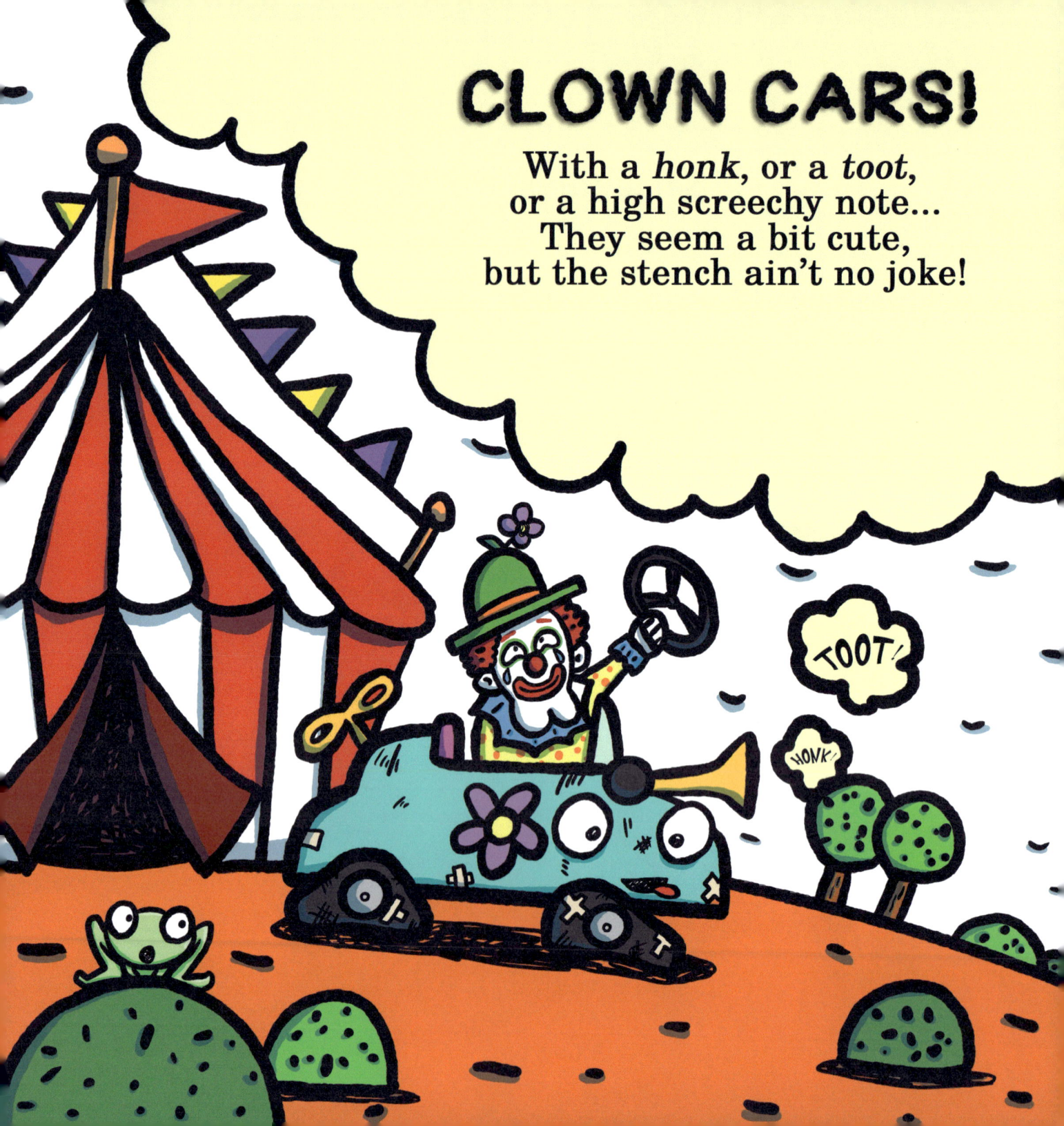

With a *honk*, or a *toot*,
or a high screechy note...
They seem a bit cute,
but the stench ain't no joke!

Some farts are like...

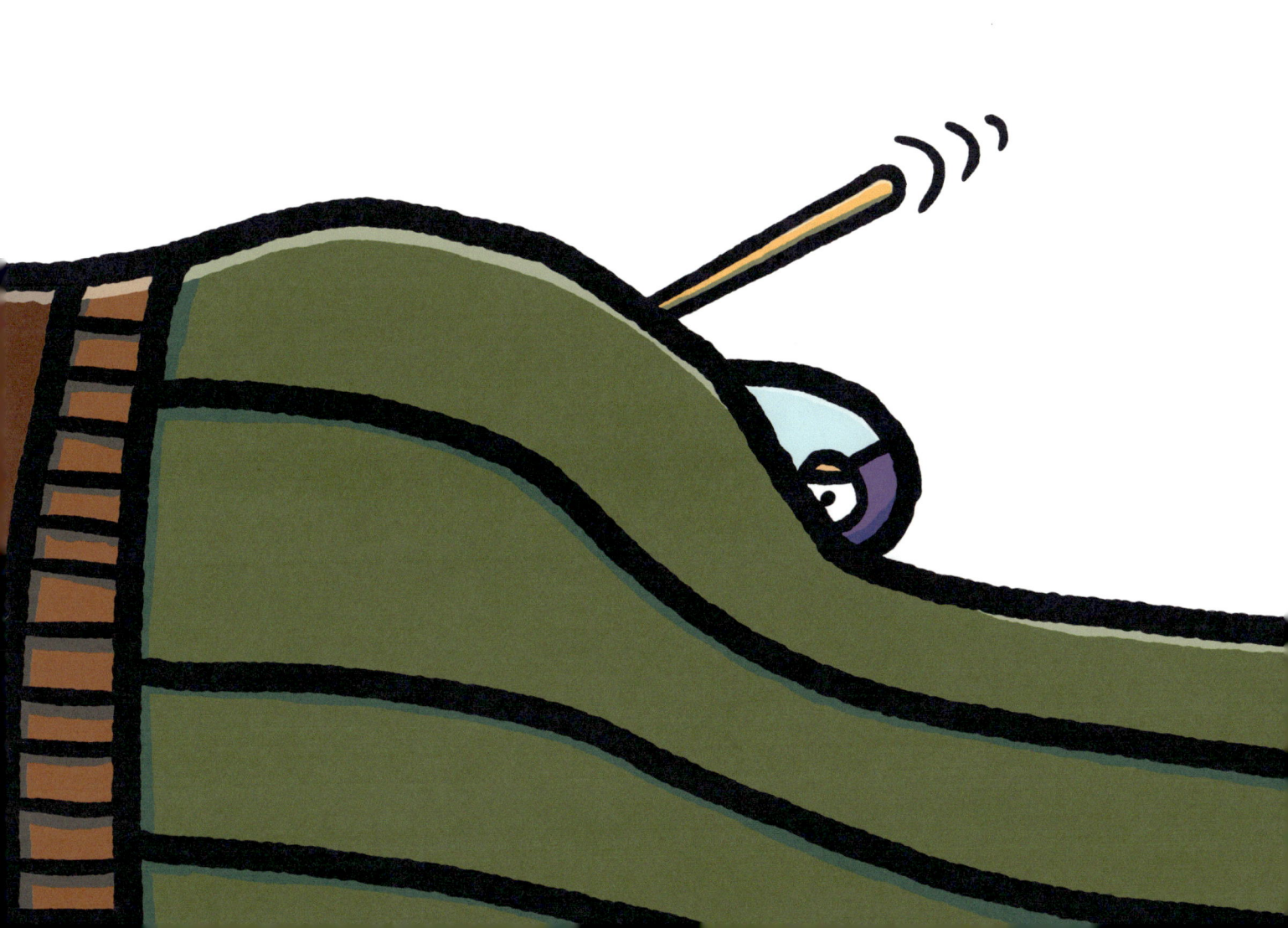

HELICOPTERS!

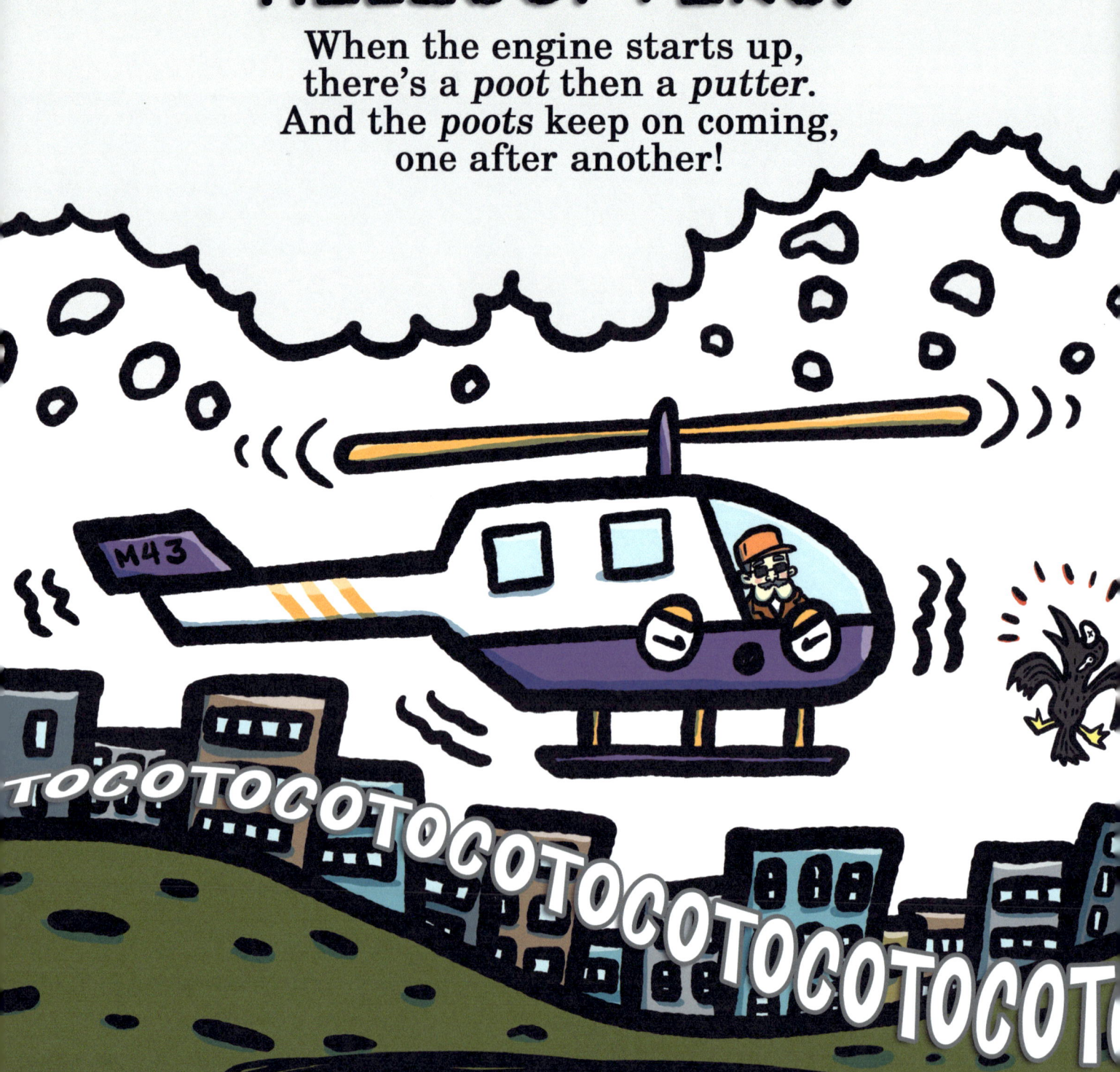

When the engine starts up,
there's a *poot* then a *putter*.
And the *poots* keep on coming,
one after another!

TOCOTOCOTOCOTOCOTOCOTOCOT

Some farts are like...

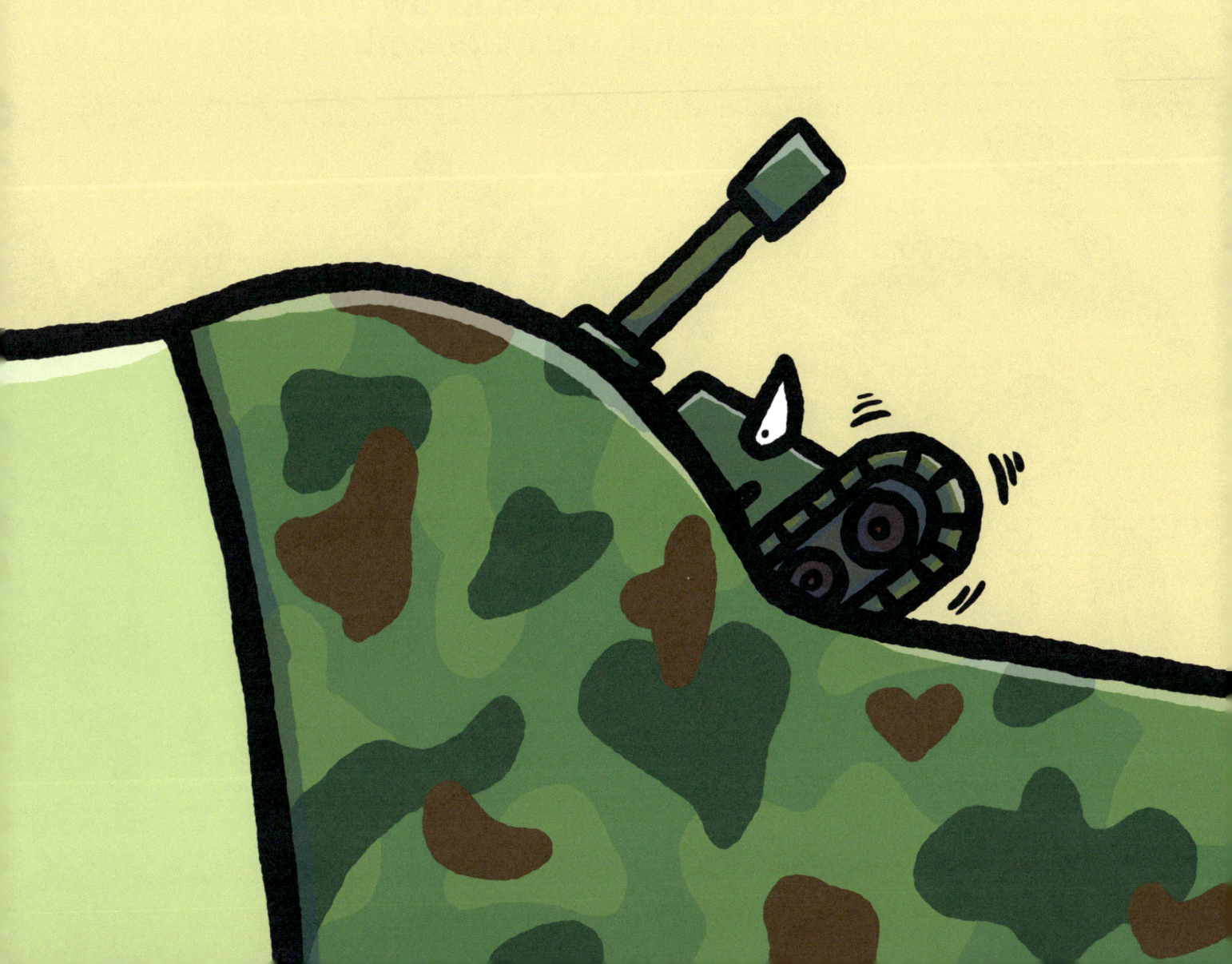

TANKS!

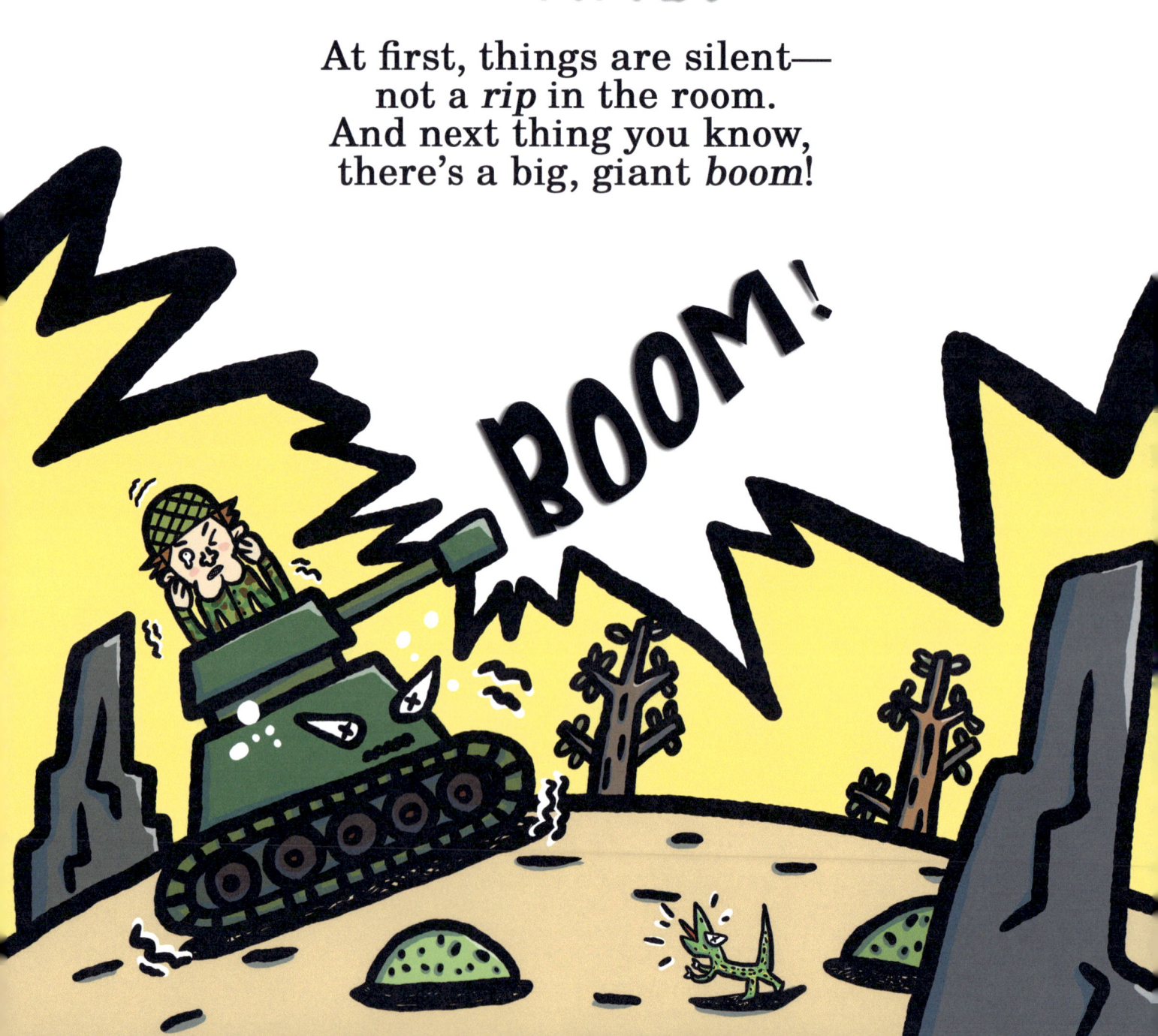

At first, things are silent—
not a *rip* in the room.
And next thing you know,
there's a big, giant *boom*!

BOOM!

Some farts are like...

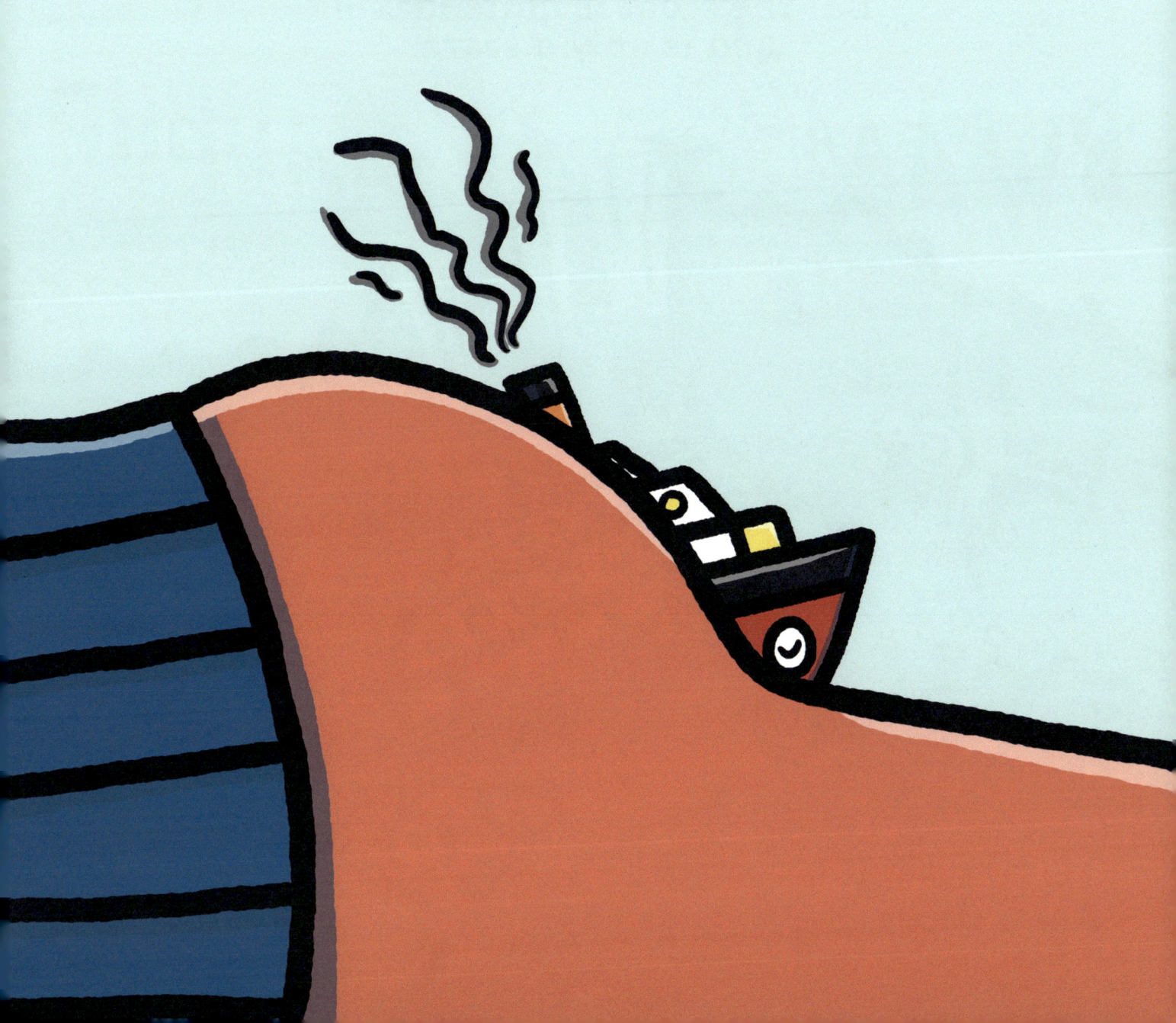

SHIPS!

Unseen and unknown,
a deep sound fills the air.
But the scent is quite lacking
and is only a scare.

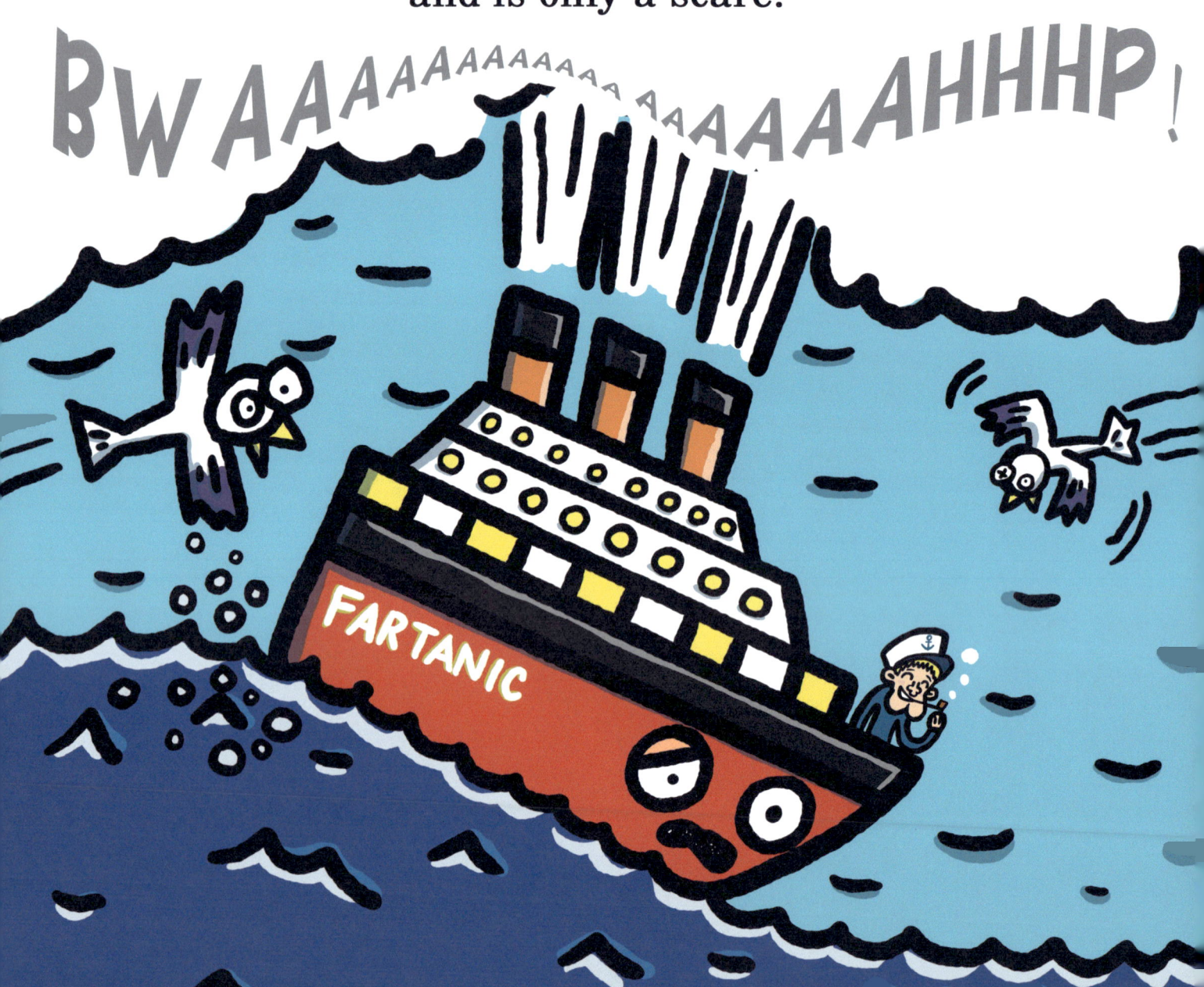

BWAAAAAAAAAAAAAAAAAAAHHHP!

FARTANIC

Some farts are like...

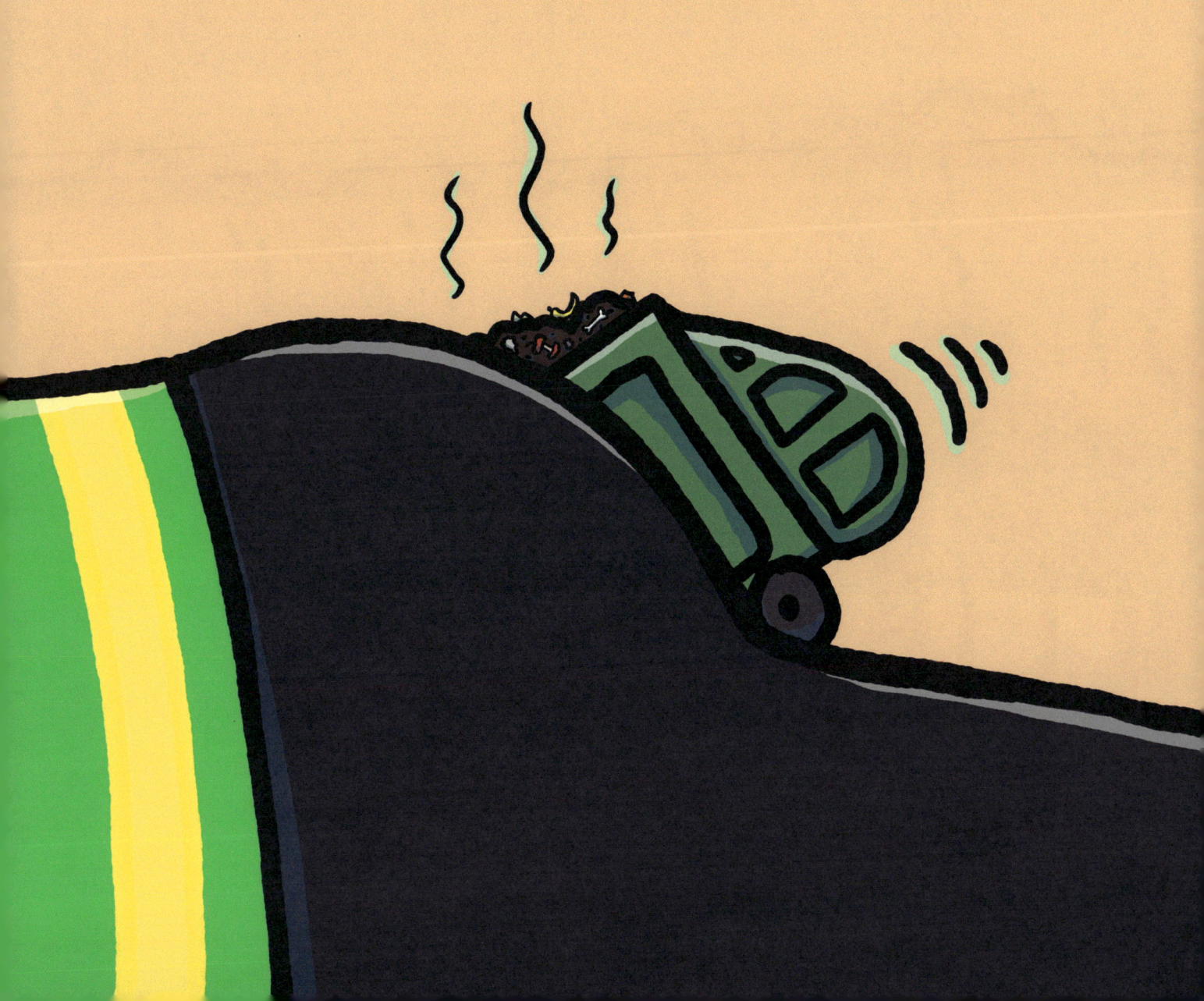

DUMP TRUCKS!

Oh! The fumes reek so bad that you hardly can breathe! The stink stays in your nose even after you leave.

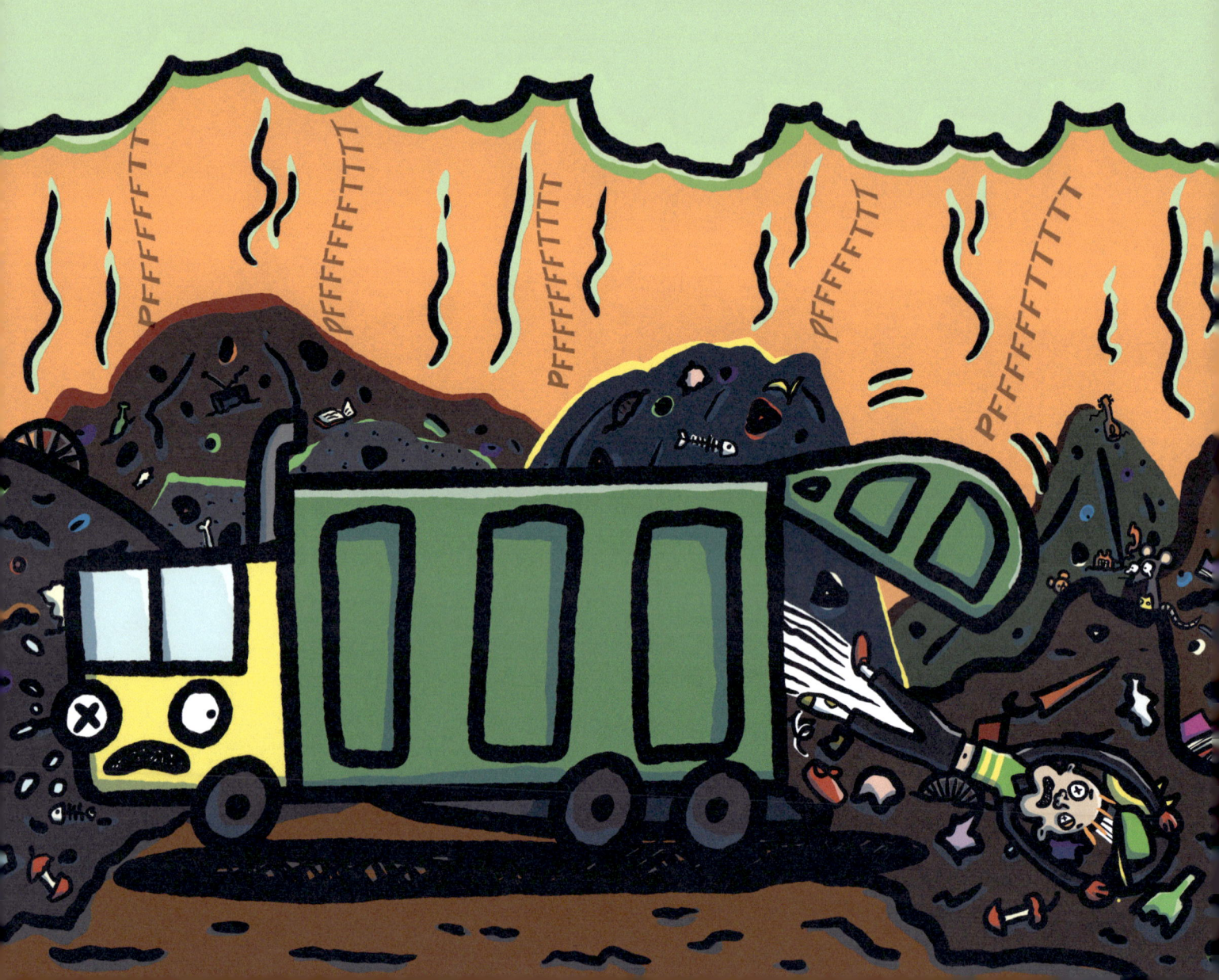

Some farts are like...

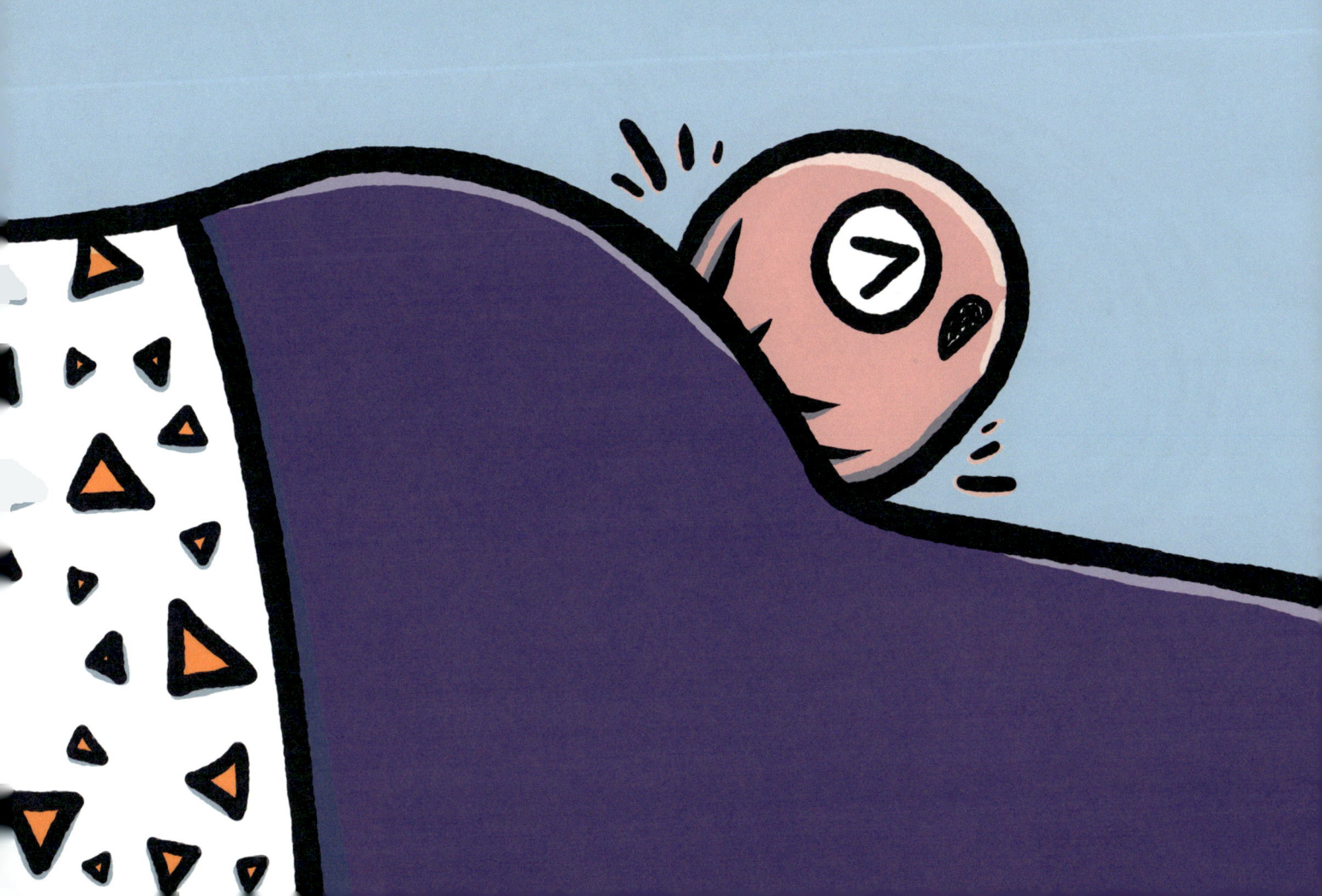

BALLOONS!

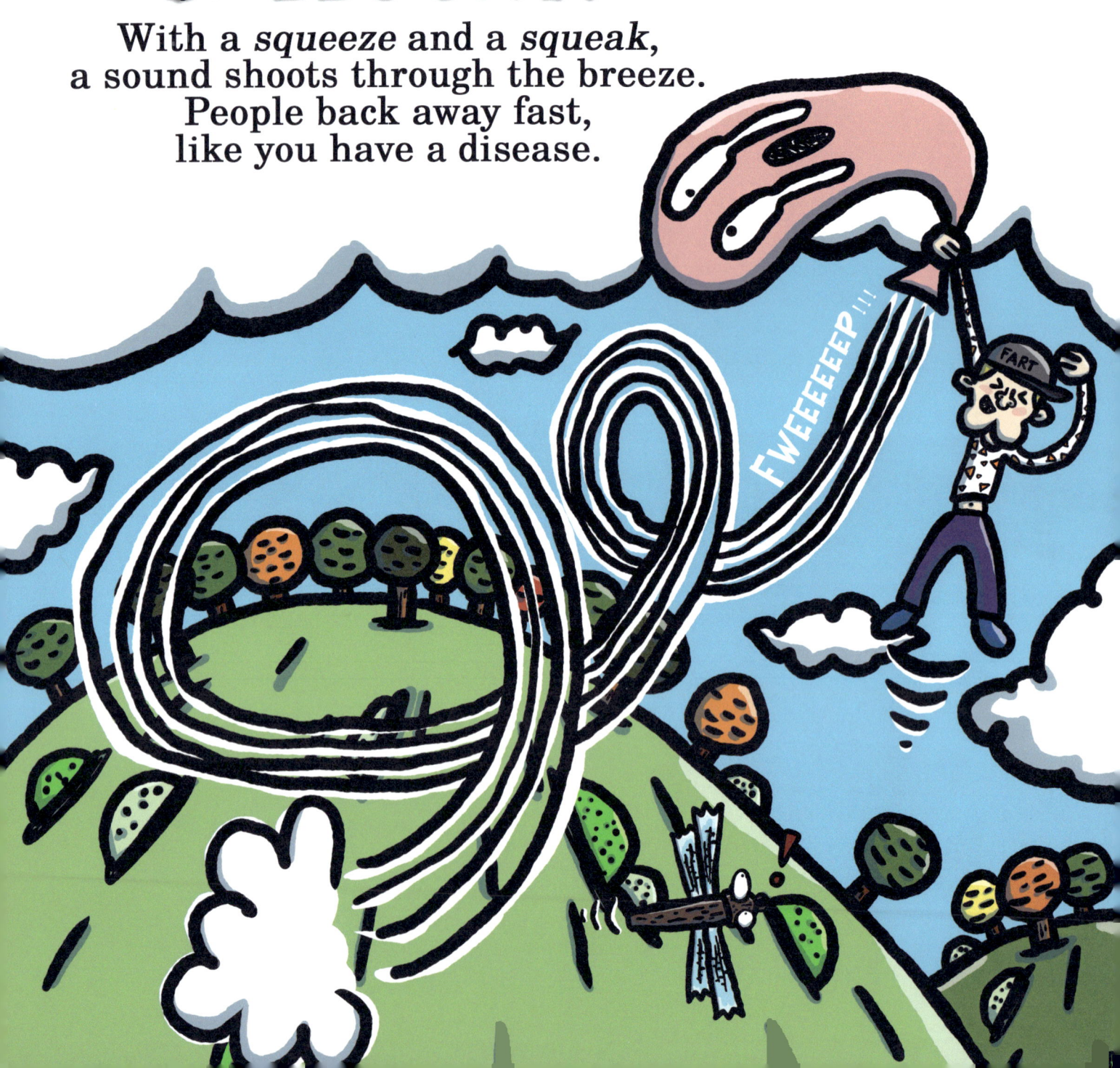

With a *squeeze* and a *squeak*,
a sound shoots through the breeze.
People back away fast,
like you have a disease.

Some farts are like...

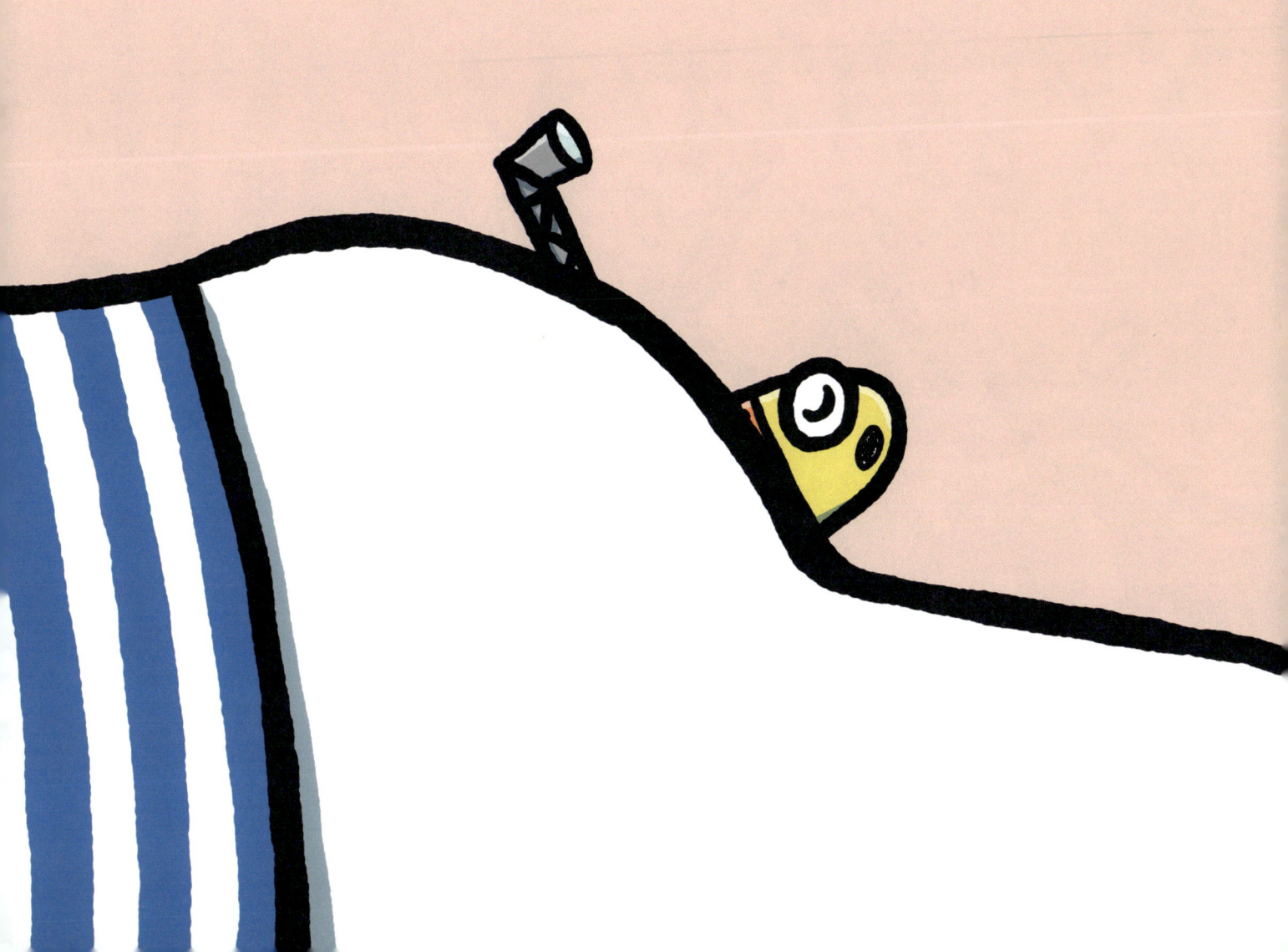

SUBMARINES!

With a *splish* and a *splash*,
you know something's come out.
Run home and get changed
before others find out!

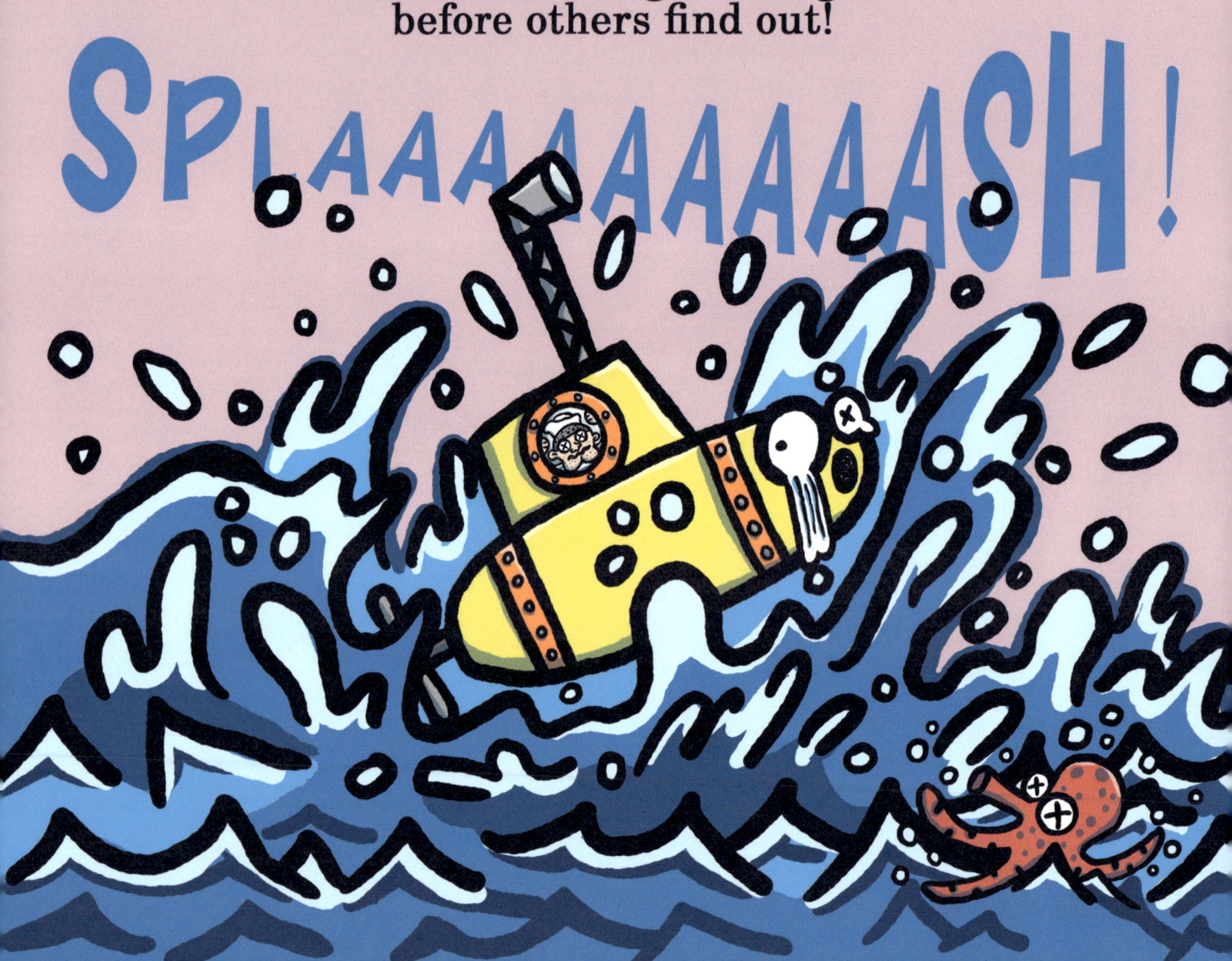

SPLAAAAAAAAAASH!

Some farts are like...

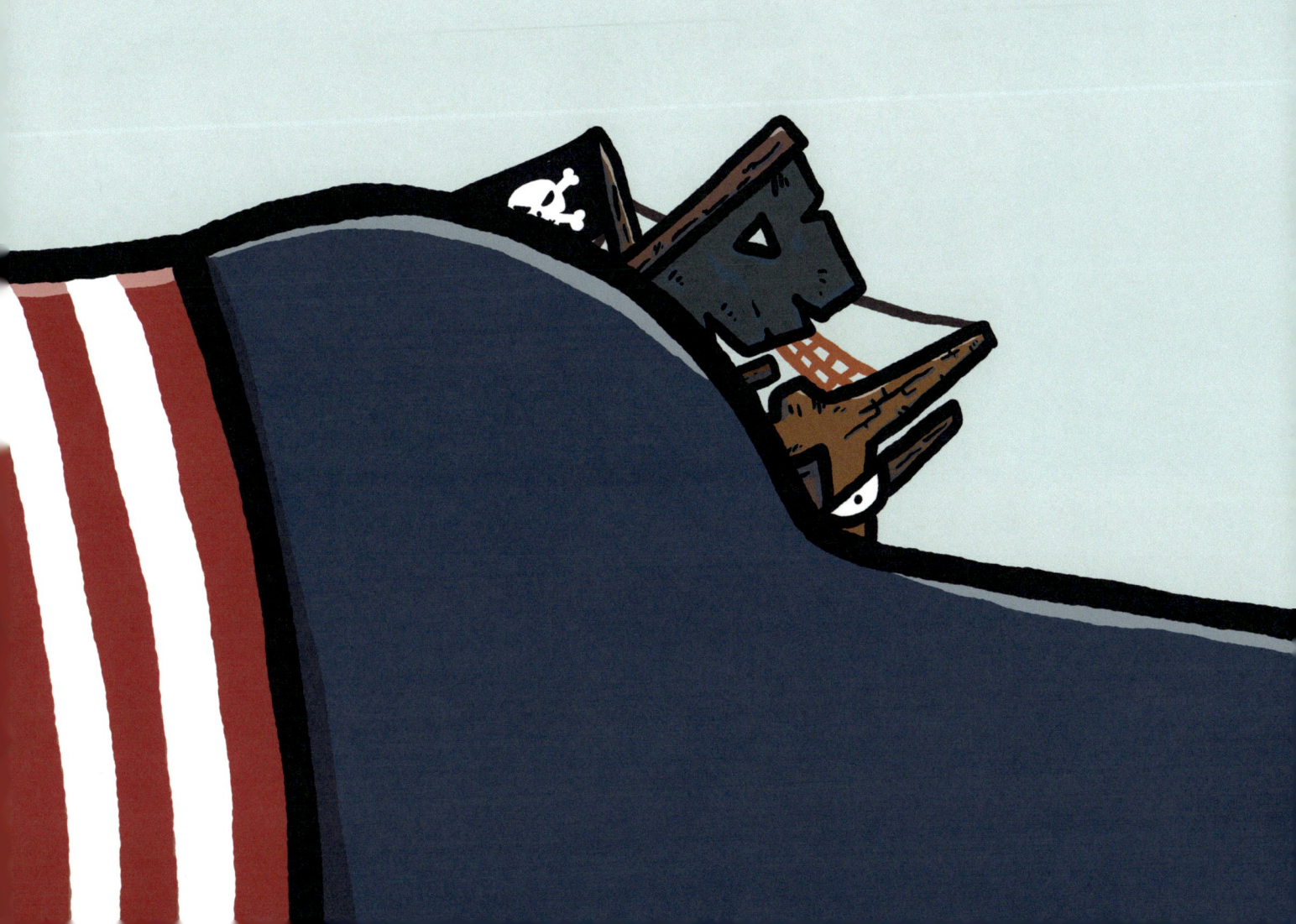

GHOST SHIPS!

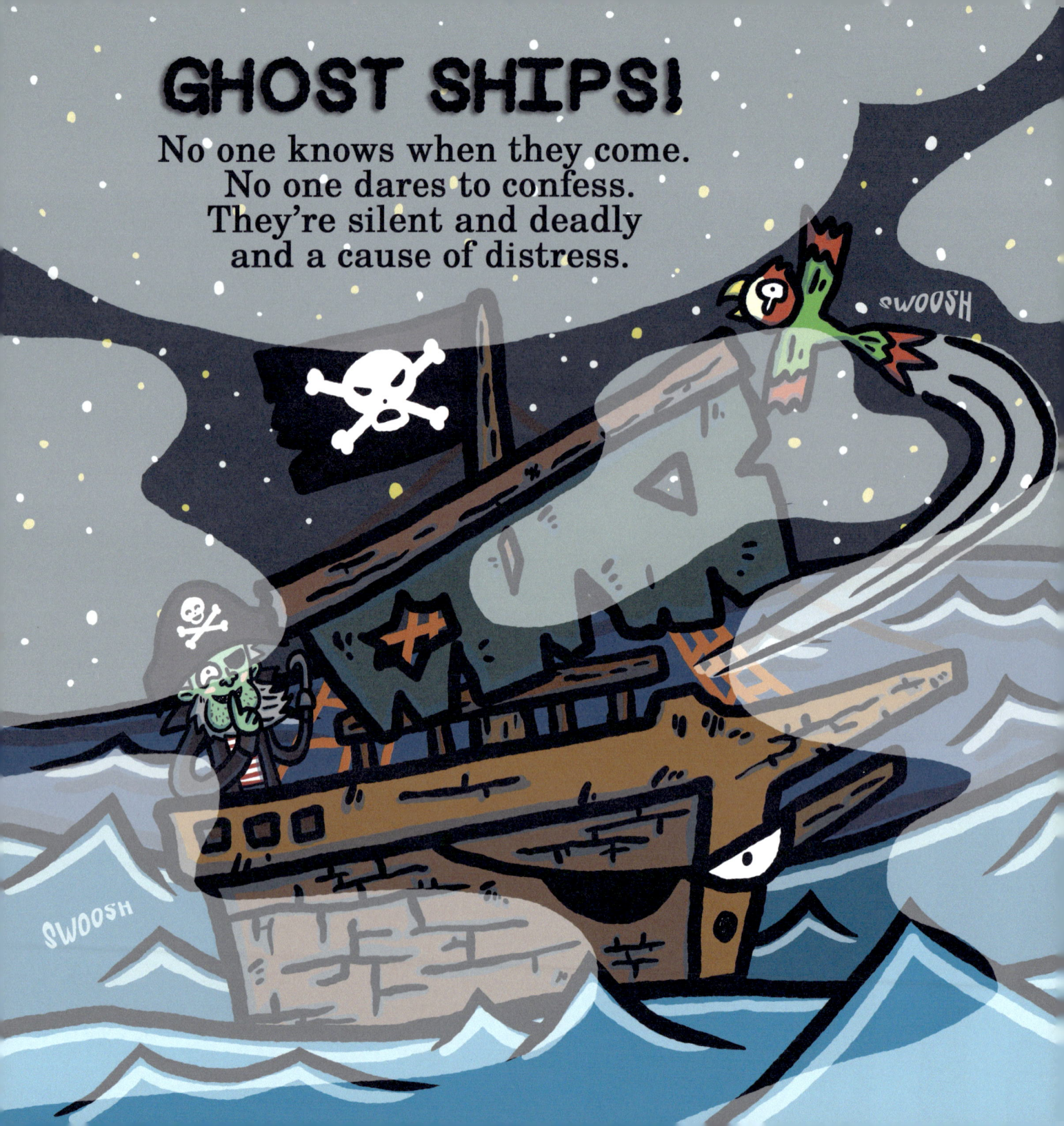

No one knows when they come.
No one dares to confess.
They're silent and deadly
and a cause of distress.

Some farts are like...

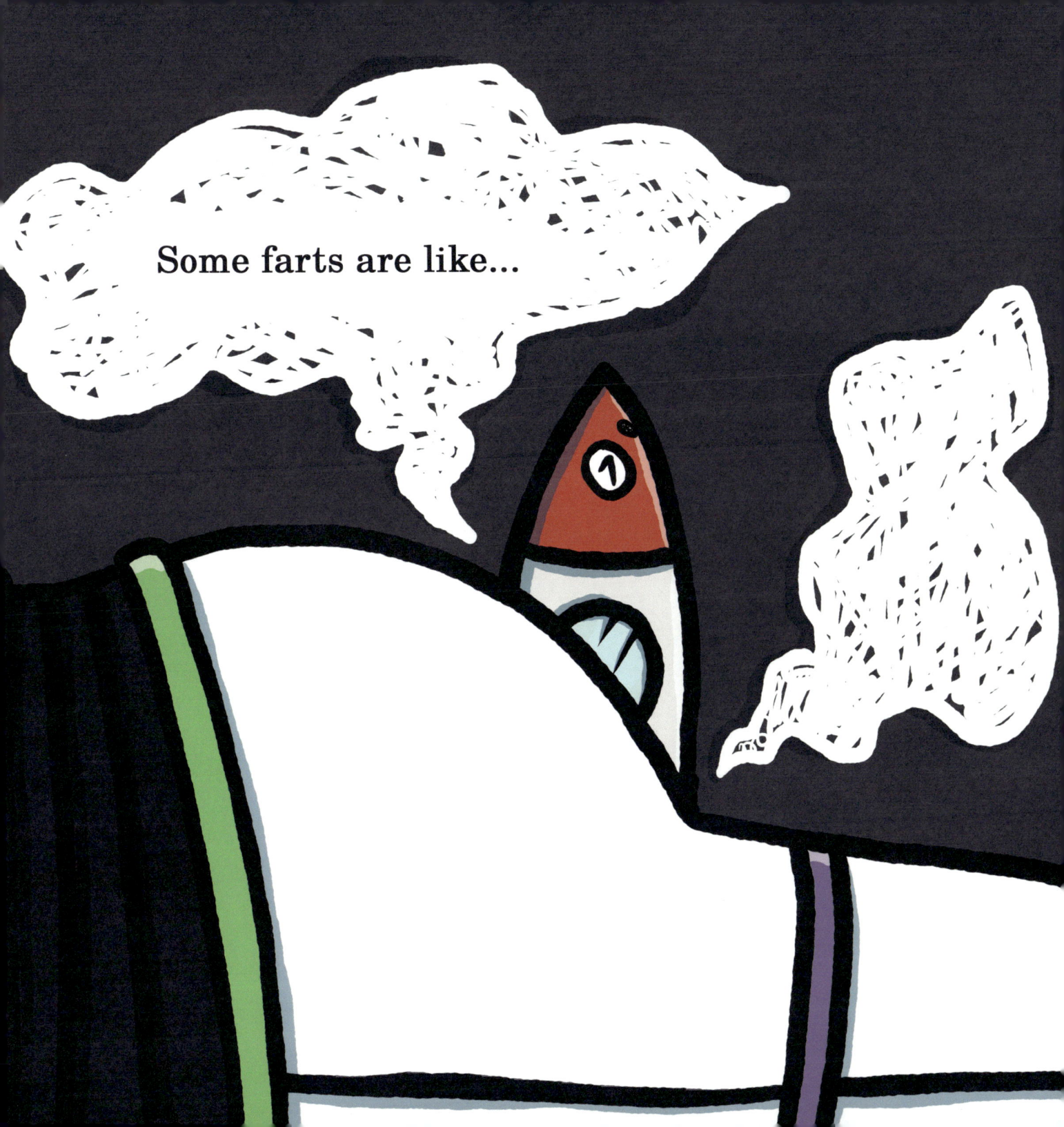

ROCKETS!

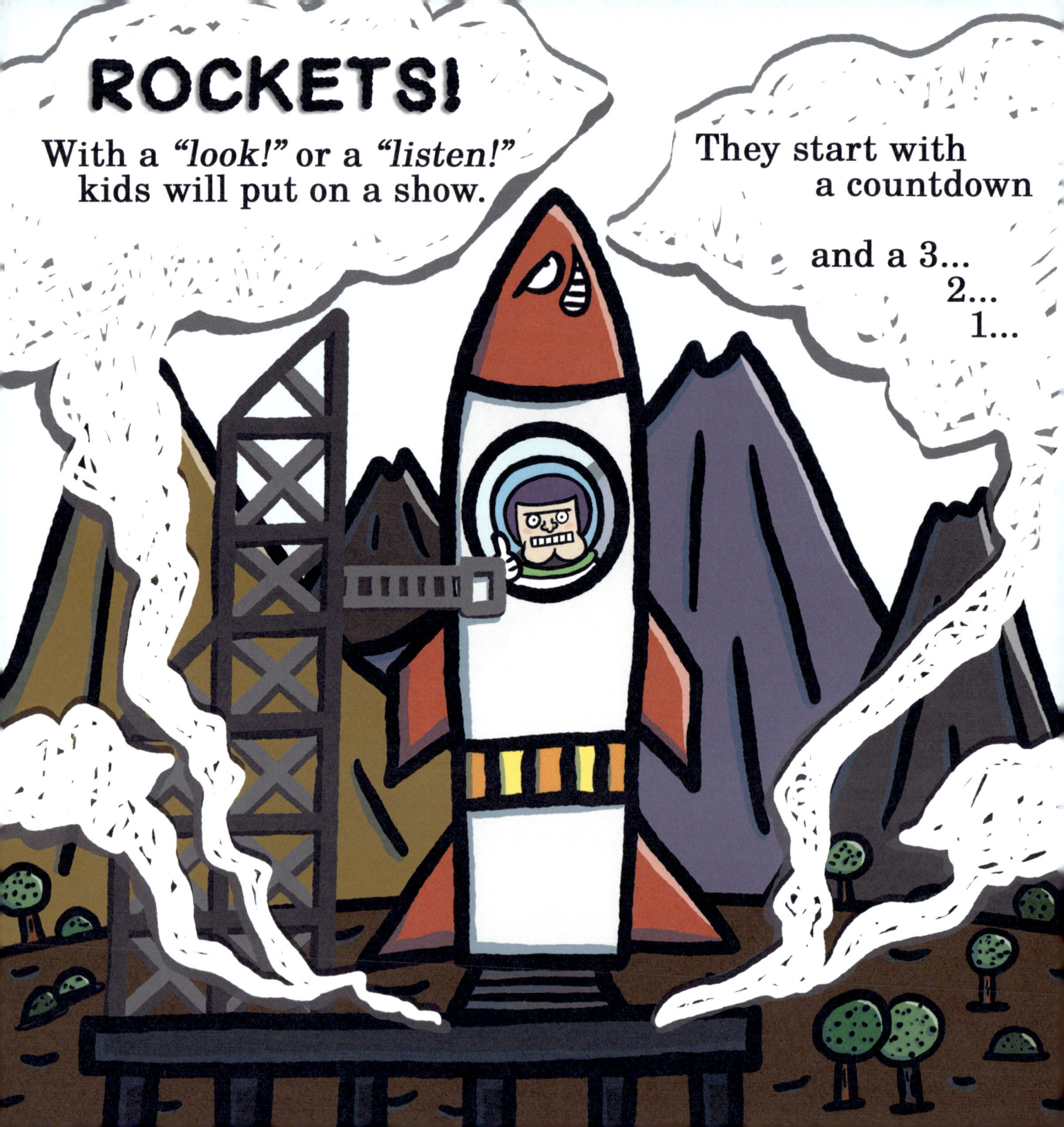

With a *"look!"* or a *"listen!"* kids will put on a show.

They start with a countdown and a 3... 2... 1...

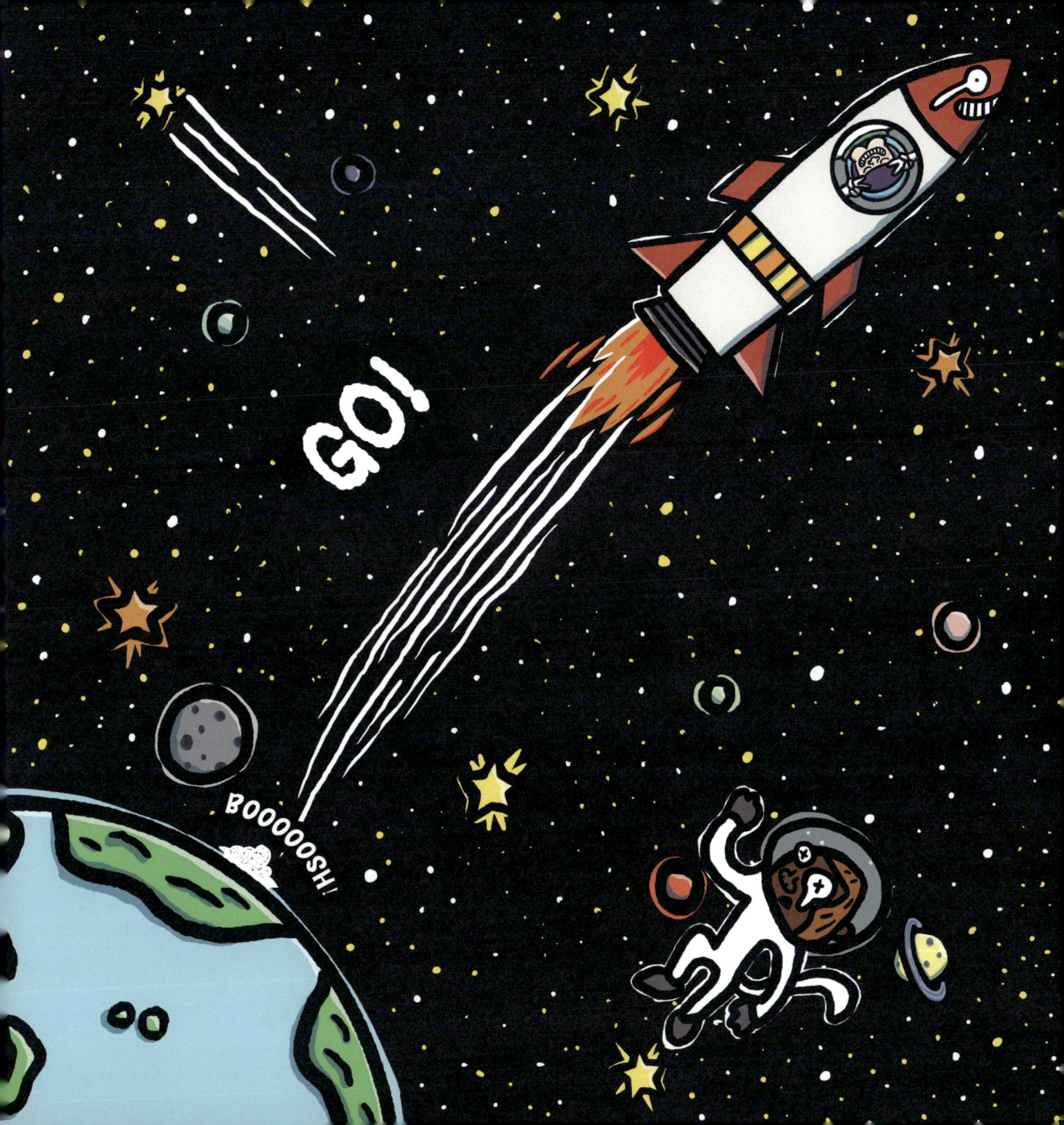

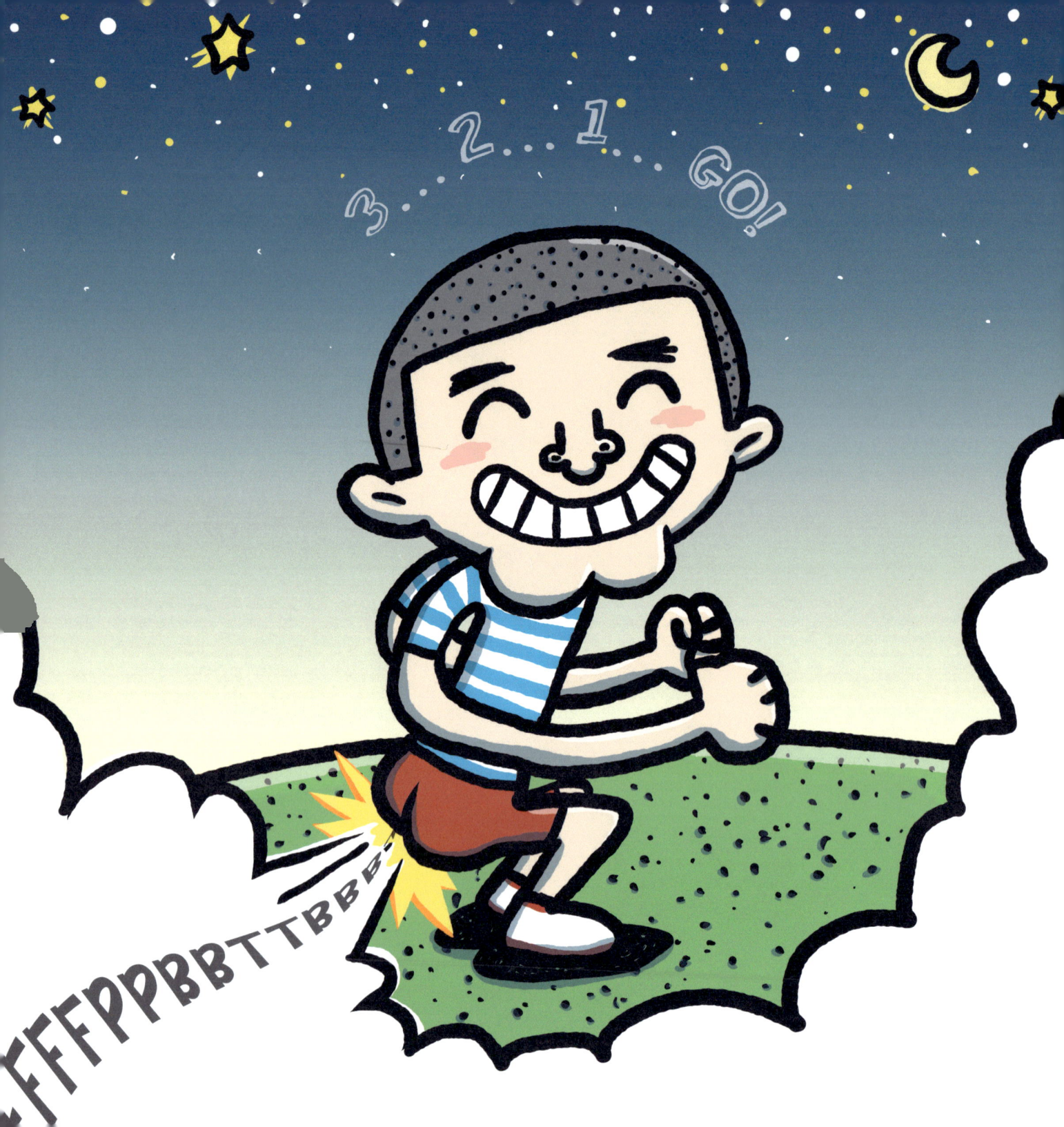

Some farts are like...

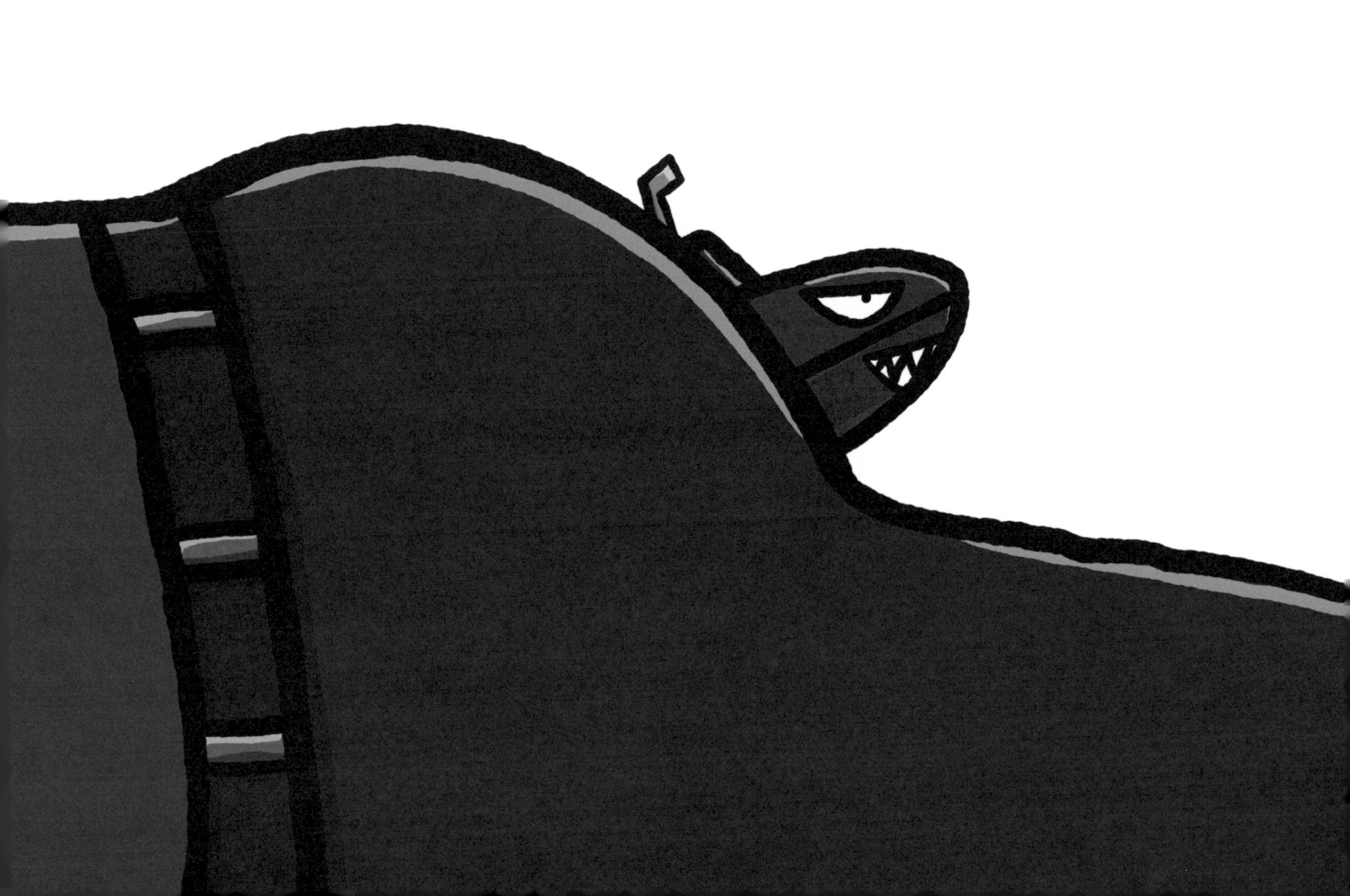

TORPEDOS!

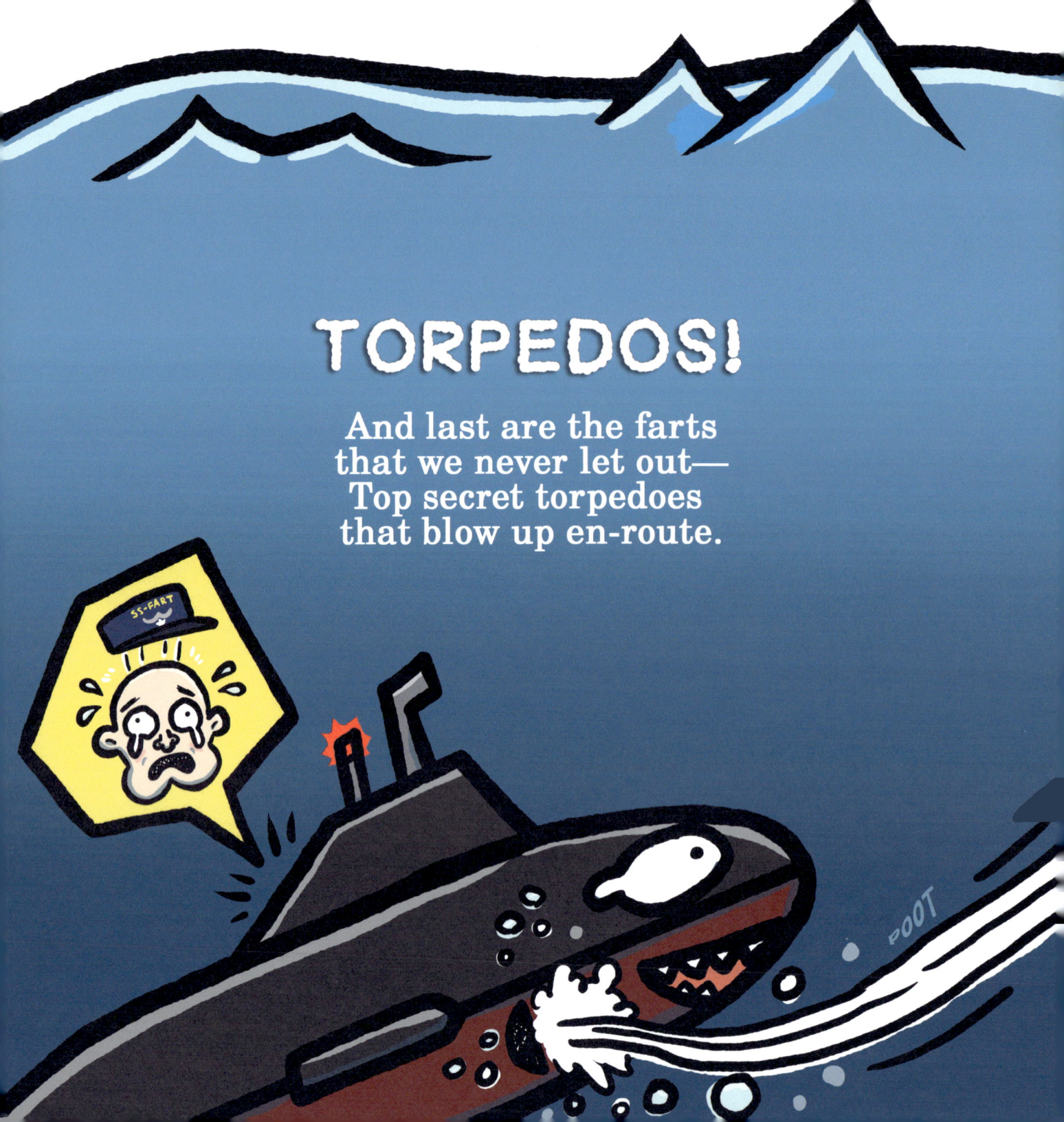

And last are the farts that we never let out—
Top secret torpedoes that blow up en-route.

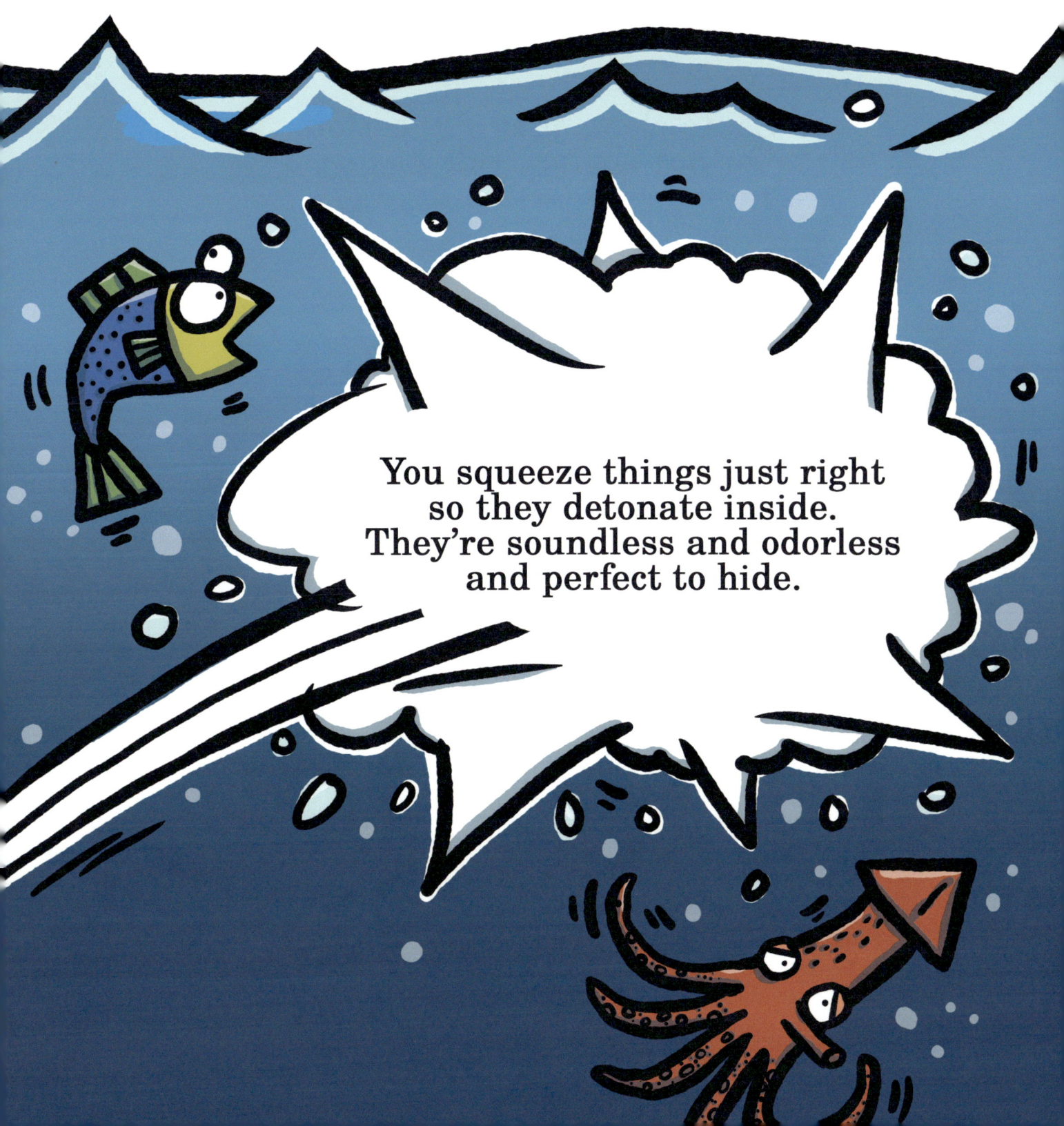

You squeeze things just right
so they detonate inside.
They're soundless and odorless
and perfect to hide.

So, to close, just a question,
for our rhyme ends at last:

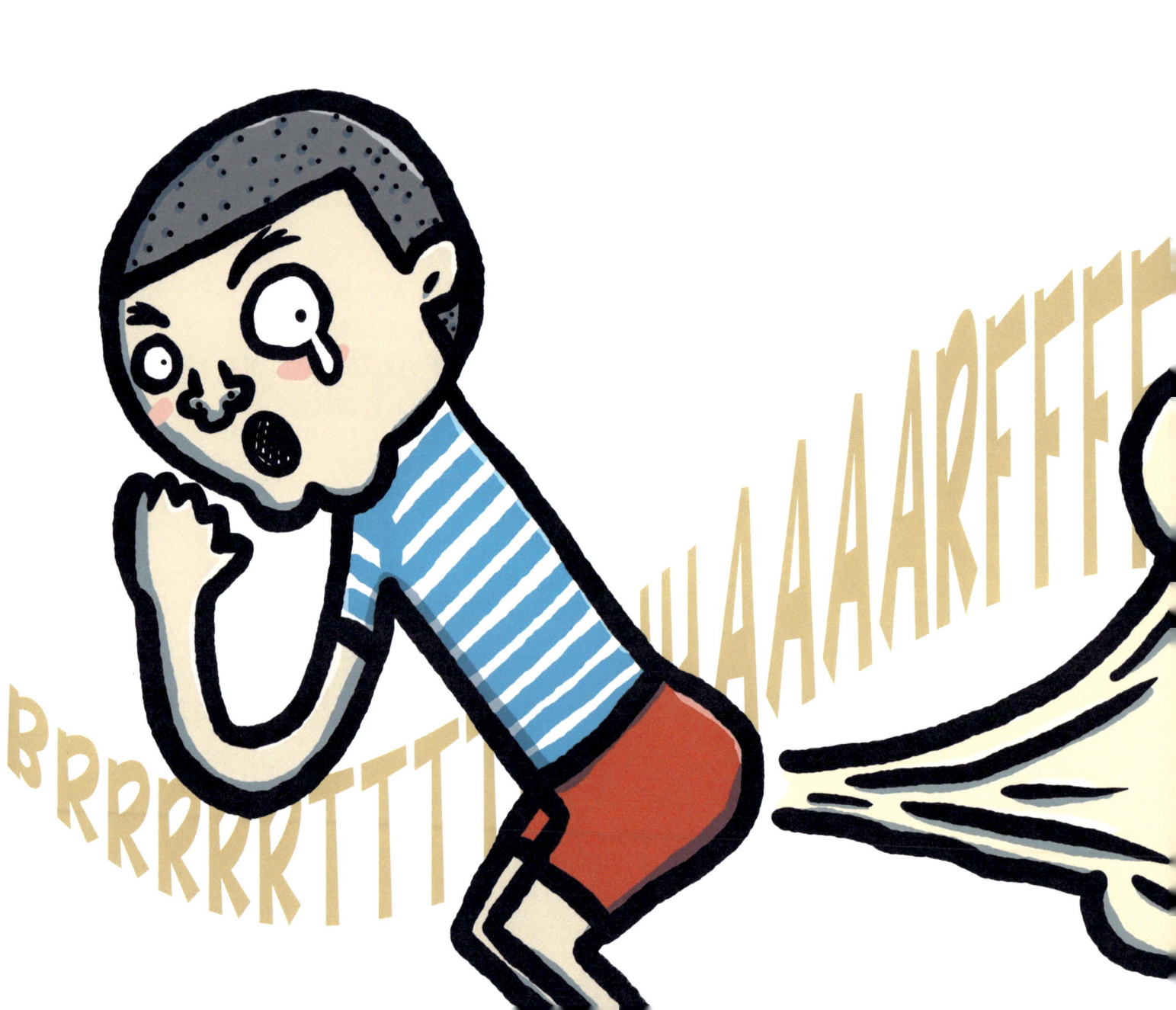

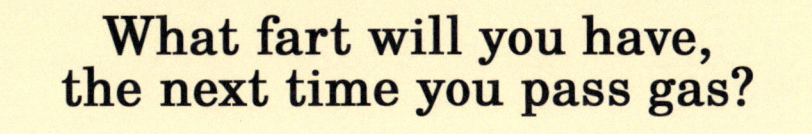

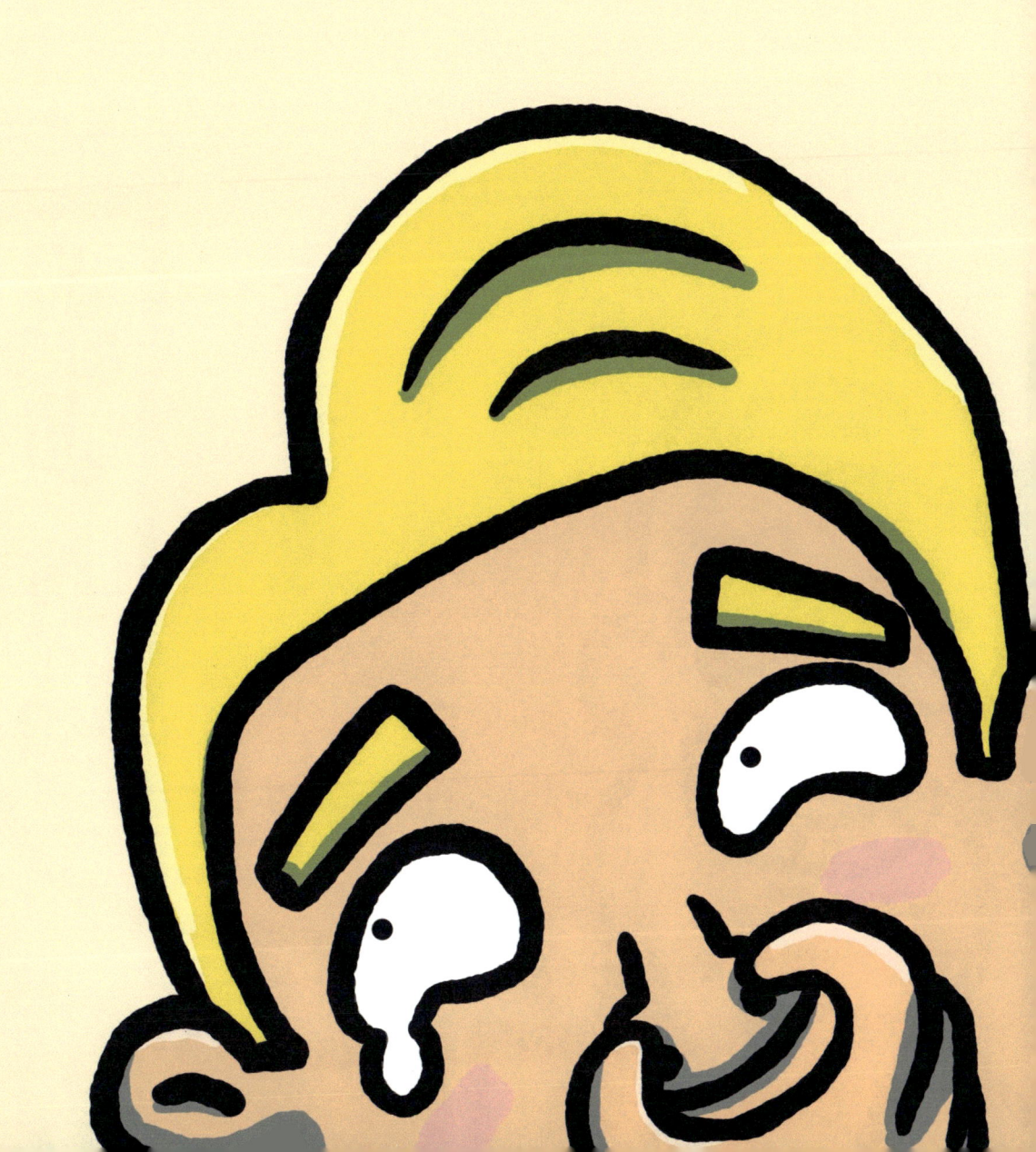

What fart will you have, the next time you pass gas?

Now, before I finish, I just want to tell you a few facts about our foul-smelling friends.

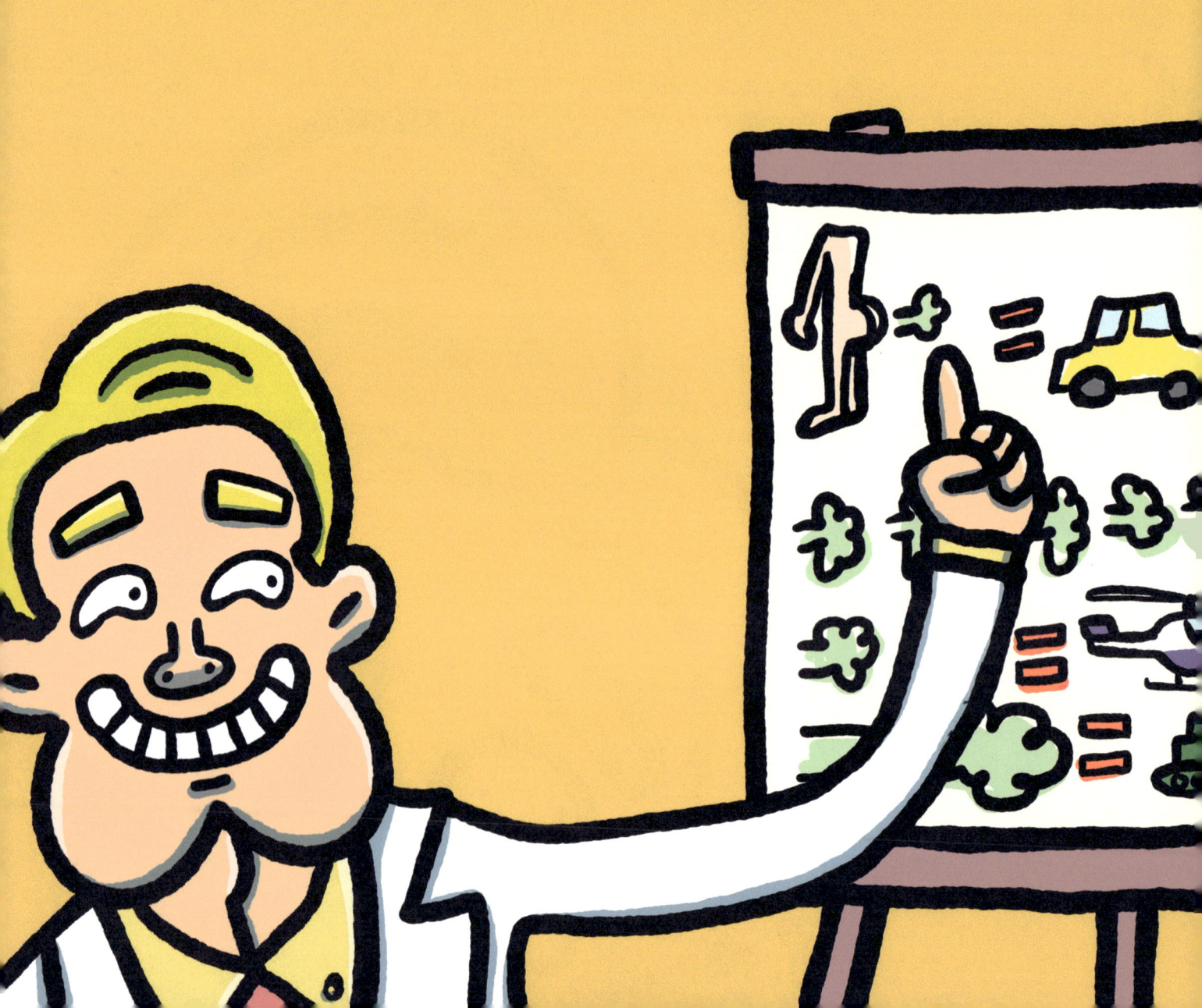

First, where do farts come from?

When we eat and digest food, gas forms inside our intestines.

Additional gas enters into our bodies from swallowing air when we chew, eat, and drink.

Drinking carbonated drinks add even more gas into our bodies!

When there is too much gas built-up, our bodies push it out in the form of a fart.

Some good news though—usually only 1% of our farts actually smell!

PBBBTTT

The rest of the 99% are made out of odorless (non-stinky) gas.

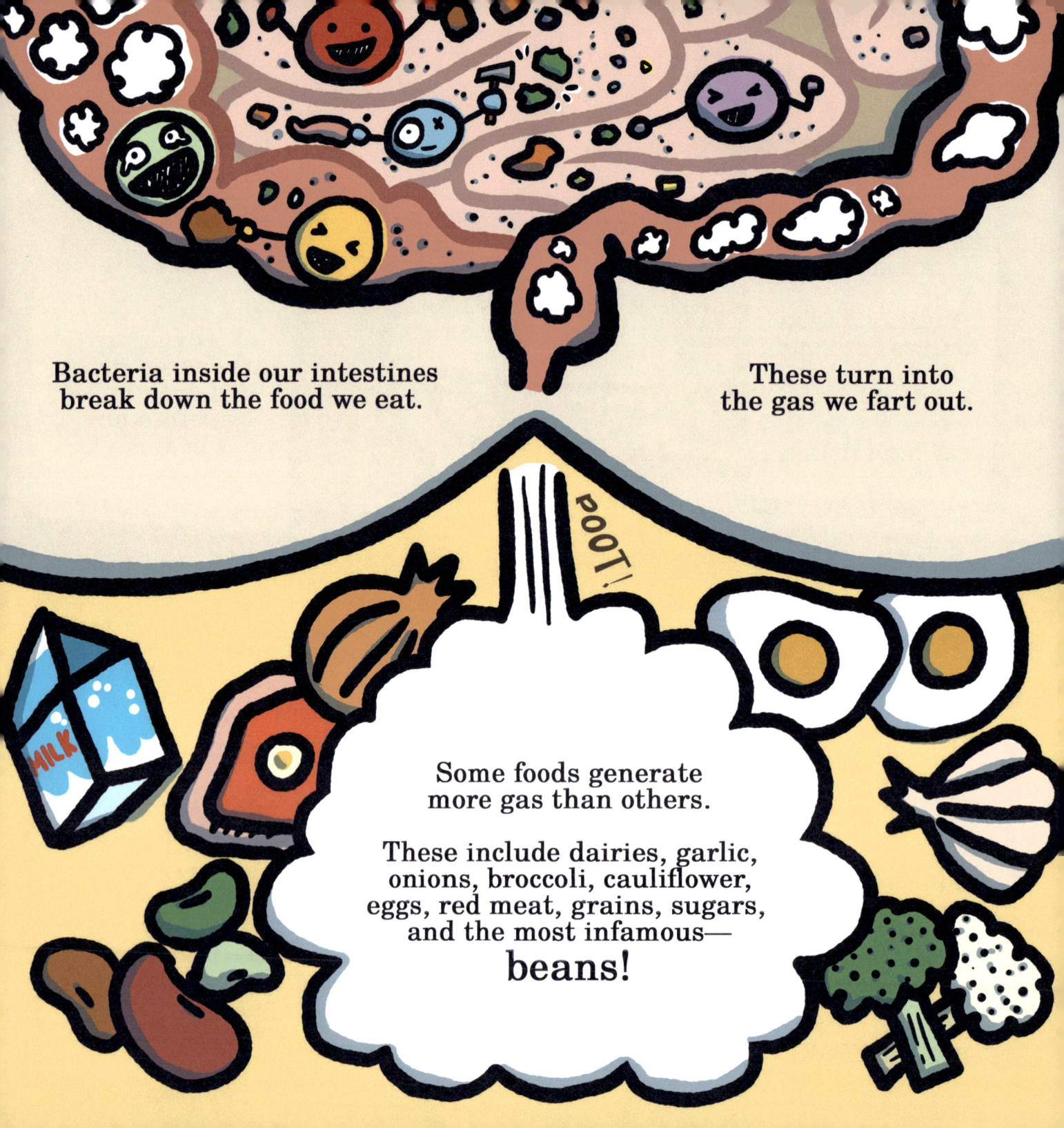

Bacteria inside our intestines break down the food we eat.

These turn into the gas we fart out.

POOT!

Some foods generate more gas than others.

These include dairies, garlic, onions, broccoli, cauliflower, eggs, red meat, grains, sugars, and the most infamous—
beans!

We fart between 12-25 times a day.
That's a whole lot of gas.

This equals to between 0.6 to 1.8 liters a day—enough to fill up a medium-sized balloon!

(Also, a fun fact: we fart more when we sleep!)

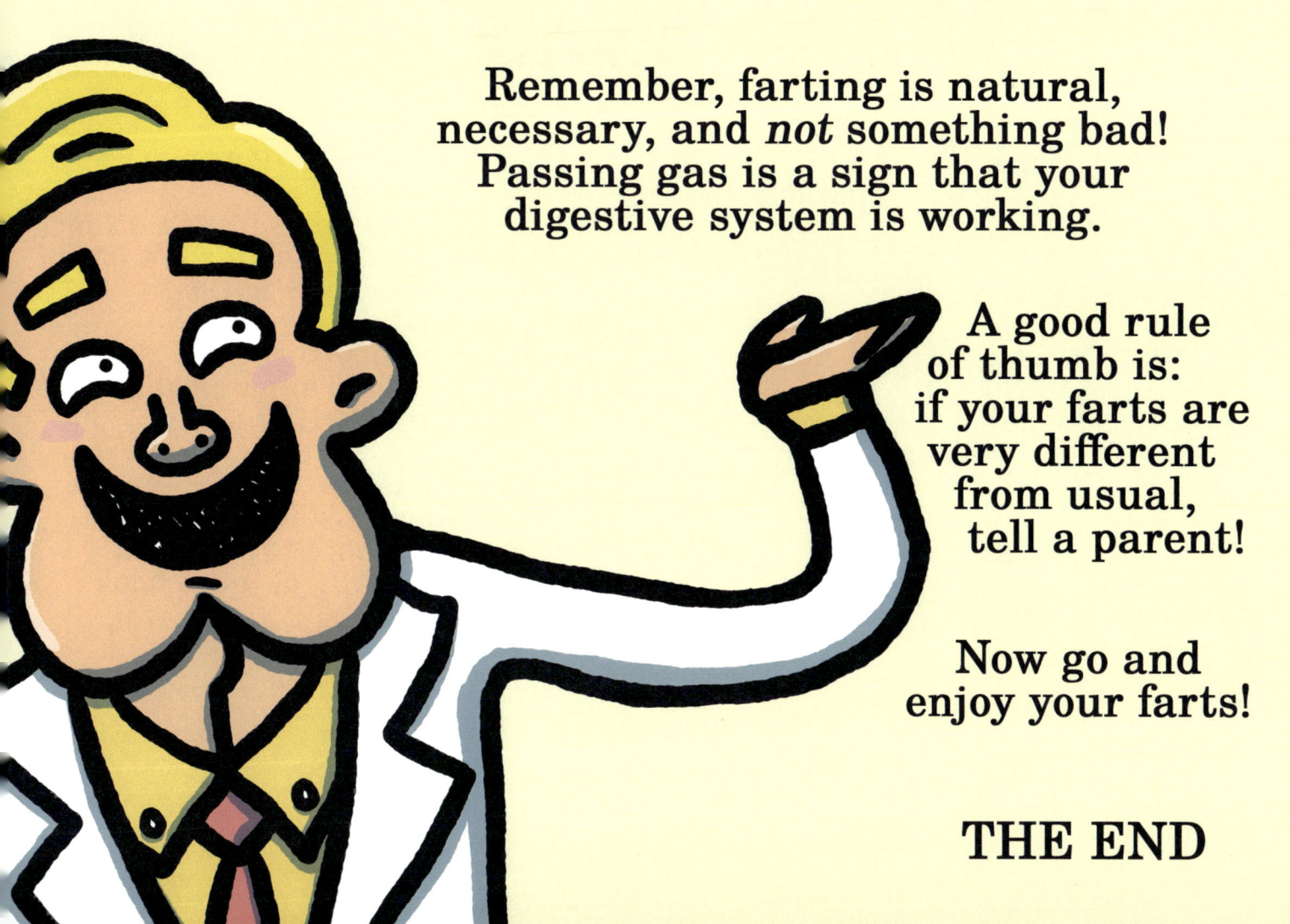

Remember, farting is natural, necessary, and *not* something bad! Passing gas is a sign that your digestive system is working.

A good rule of thumb is: if your farts are very different from usual, tell a parent!

Now go and enjoy your farts!

THE END

The Fart Book
A Book for Children to Enjoy and Learn About Farts

ISBN 978-1-952343-00-1

Copyright © 2020
Mark Bacera and
Rounded Specs Publishing

www.roundedspecspublishing.com
FB.me/roundedspecspublishing
Instagram: @roundedspecspublishing

Authors love reviews!
To leave one, visit:
www.amazon.com/dp/B0876QB839

About the Author

Mark Bacera is a bestselling author and released his first children's book called The Poo Poo Book (also the first book in the Bewildering Body series) in 2018. Since then, he has followed that up with several other titles.

The author lives in western Japan with his wonderful wife and daughter who also participate in the creative process and making of these books.

Amazon Author Page:
http://www.amazon.com/mark-bacera/e/B0198eht0m

Email:
mark@roundedspecspublishing.com

Other Books

By Mark

The Poo Poo Book
The Belly Button Book
The Booger Book
The Stinky Feet Book
The Ear Wax Book
The Sweat Book
The Tear Book
The Spit Book
Baby Poop
A Naughty Kid's Christmas
I'm an Alien-Vampire and I'm Proud

By Rounded Specs

A Day With Mae
Ame the Cat
Ame Goes to Japan
Ame Goes to Hawaii
Ame Goes to the North Pole
Ame Goes to Egypt
Ame Goes to the Zoo
Ame's First Christmas
Ame's Cafe
Fashionable Animals
What in the World Could it Be?

Please note that some of the above titles have yet to be published. To support us and be notified when new books are in the works and released, send us an email at info@roundedspecspublishing.com

Made in United States
Troutdale, OR
08/19/2024